Caring and Competent Caregivers

Caring & Competent Caregivers

Robert M. Moroney, Ph.D.

Paul R. Dokecki, Ph.D.

John J. Gates, Ph.D.

Kelly Noser Haynes, M.A.

J. R. Newbrough, Ph.D.

Jack A. Nottingham, Ph.D.

with contributions from:

Pam Davis, M.Ed.

David H. Haigler, Ed.D.

Anne G. McWilliams, M.S.

David L. Smith, Ph.D.

The University of Georgia Press   *Athens and London*

© 1998 by the University of Georgia Press
Athens, Georgia 30602
All rights reserved
Designed by Louise OFarrell
Set in 11/14.5 Minion by G&S Typesetters, Inc.
Printed and bound by Braun-Brumfield, Inc.

The paper in this book meets the guidelines for permanence
and durability of the Committee on Production Guidelines for
Book Longevity of the Council on Library Resources.

Printed in the United States of America

02 01 00 99 98   C   5 4 3 2 1

02 01 00 99 98   P   5 4 3 2 1

Library of Congress Cataloging in Publication Data
Caring and competent caregivers / Robert M. Moroney, general editor.
   p. cm.
Includes bibliographical references and index.
ISBN 0-8203-1951-1 (alk. paper). — ISBN 0-8203-1952-x (pbk. : alk. paper)
1. Caregivers—United States. 2. Caregivers—Government policy—United
States. I. Moroney, Robert, 1936–
HV40.42.C37 1998
362.4—dc21   97-19748
British Library Cataloging in Publication Data available

This book is dedicated to a remarkable group of people who were instrumental in the creation of the Rosalynn Carter Institute and, through their service as members of the institute's board of directors, supported its growth. These visionaries were Charles Crisp and Russell Thomas Jr. of the Charles L. Mix Foundation, Arthur Cheokas, Anne Hale, Jack Moses (deceased), Betty Pope, and William H. Capitan, former president of Georgia Southwestern State University. America's caregivers are better acknowledged, understood, and served thanks to the altruism of these Georgians.

Contents

Foreword

As we near the close of the twentieth century, we are fortunate to have this very timely book appear. While it describes the remarkable progress of the past hundred years, it deals with the formidable human problems accompanying that progress.

Let me illustrate: life expectancy at birth has gone from forty-eight years at the turn of the century to seventy-six years now; the acute infectious diseases of childhood have been virtually eliminated; mortality from heart disease and stroke has declined by 30 and 60 percent, respectively, over the past thirty years; and we have, for the first time, begun to observe a decline in mortality from cancer.

The great revolution in biology since World War II has resulted in new technologies that have focused on curing disease. Yet we should observe that our great progress has largely been the result of the public health applications of our knowledge: safe food and water supplies, improved sanitation, immunizations, better nutrition, exercise, and reduction in cigarette smoking.

This is not to disparage our progress in medical knowledge and its focus on curing. Rather, all progress is accompanied by new problems. Therein lies the importance of this book. It is an important step in redressing the imbalance between curing and caring.

A few facts illustrate the problem:

∾ Chronic conditions are the leading cause of illness, disability, and death in the United States today.

∾ Almost 100 million Americans have one or more chronic conditions.

∾ More than 40 million people are limited in their daily activities by chronic conditions—and the numbers of people so affected are expected to increase dramatically in the coming decades.

∞ People are living longer with chronic conditions than ever before.

∞ Chronic conditions cost the economy $470 billion (in 1990 dollars) in direct medical costs in 1995 and more than $230 billion in lost productivity.

The authors point out that as a society we have not yet adapted to these changes. Since Americans pride themselves on living in a caring society, these issues must move higher on our national agenda. We have some evidence that this may be happening through the passage of the Americans with Disabilities Act (1990), but that is not enough. The efforts by and large are disorganized, fragmented, and sporadic. In part this is due to the complexity of the problems. No single agency, institution, or discipline has all the requisite skills and resources.

This volume can serve as a guidebook to deal with this complexity. Because improved care depends on the capacity of caregivers, they are central to the text. From involvement of family members, community support groups, and agencies to the many professions dealing with caregiving, the authors deal with the short- and long-term issues involved in improving services. They are especially insightful in defining the obstacles to a more effective care system. And they never lose sight of the intensely personal issues involved in caregiving and receiving.

As a society we stand on the threshold of striking a balance between our curing and caring. These authors are helping us to find our way.

Julius B. Richmond, M.D.
John D. MacArthur Professor of Health Policy, Emeritus
Harvard Medical School

Preface

My book *Helping Yourself Help Others: A Book for Caregivers* was written to assist family members and friends who are dealing with the challenge of providing care to someone with a long-term physical or mental illness. I drew upon personal experiences with caregiving in my own family and upon research done by the Rosalynn Carter Institute at Georgia Southwestern State University. And while my book also is beneficial to professionals, I thought that another one more specifically directed to those who have dedicated their careers to caring for others was needed. Such a book, I believed, should also explore the issues related to preparing people for work in the helping professions.

Caring and Competent Caregivers fills this void. It is directed to academicians who conduct professional training programs and to diverse health care professionals who are on the front lines providing assistance to others. Incorporating philosophy, social science research, and impressionistic evidence, this book provides a basis for education and practice that is both inspirational and practical. It emphasizes the mutual stake that formal (professional) and informal (lay) caregivers have with care recipients in coping with the challenges of providing ethical and effective health care in the rapidly approaching twenty-first century. It also helps informal caregivers and consumers of services understand social policies and professional orientations that have implications for their personal well-being.

I am grateful to the authors, most of whom are associated with the Rosalynn Carter Institute, who have produced this volume. Their diversity, willingness to collaborate unselfishly for a protracted period of time, and vision blended with pragmatism are models of what the caregiving process should be. Hopefully, this book will enhance the vital contribution that America's caregivers make to our lives.

Rosalynn Carter
President of the Board of Directors
Rosalynn Carter Institute of Georgia Southwestern State University

Acknowledgments

The authors gratefully acknowledge the financial support received from the Charles L. Mix Memorial Fund and The Pew Charitable Trusts, which made this book possible. Helping in another way, but important as well, were numerous members of the National Quality Caregiving Coalition (NQCC), who offered advice, wisdom, and support. Appreciation is also expressed to Craig Lichtenwalner, M.D., and Jim Dodd, Ph.D., members of the West Central Georgia Caregivers' Network (CARE-NET), for reviewing and commenting on the initial draft of the manuscript. Beth Morris, administrative secretary at the Rosalynn Carter Institute, assisted in getting the manuscript in a suitable form for submission. Finally, we thank the hundreds of informal and formal caregivers who took part in the CARE-NET study that is quoted extensively in the text. We hope this volume will become a testament to the significance of their caregiving—and how the process could be improved.

Caring and Competent Caregivers

1 ᦟ   Caring and Caregiving: The Challenge We Face

This, then, is the basic pattern of caring, understood as helping the other grow: I experience the other as an extension of myself and also as independent of myself and with a need to grow; I experience the other's development as bound up with my own sense of well-being; and feel needed by it for that growing. I respond affirmatively and with devotion to the other's need guided by the direction of its growth.
—Milton Mayeroff, *On Caring*

Today, in medicine, law, psychology, and education, the goal that is coming onto center stage is implicit in the question: What kind of person do we want the clinician to be? . . . The surgeon who is a masterful craftsperson, the teacher who has mastered subject matter and pedagogical technique, the lawyer so thoroughly sophisticated about divorce law, the mental health clinician deeply knowledgeable about the tactics of influence and persuasion—in all of these instances, we hope for more than technical knowledge and skill; we hope for understanding, caring, and compassion and that sense that our symptoms and problems are not treated in isolation from what we are and need, from what we are as persons.
—Seymour Sarason, *Caring and Compassion in Clinical Practice*

IN THIS BOOK, we explore several issues that are the subject of intense debate and will continue to be of concern well into the twenty-first century. One issue involves the dynamics of *caring*: the extent to which we as individuals care for people we know and, just as important, how we as members of a nation care for those we do not know personally—the others, the strangers in our midst. But caring is only one issue. A related, more general issue is *caregiving*.

1

Caring is a special relationship to others—entailing feelings, attitudes, knowledge, and skill—in which they are treated as persons deserving of respect and helped to enhance their well-being and human development. Caregiving is the more general act of providing services and support to those in need. Caregiving, however, may or may not be caring. For example, although overmedicating an aging person in a large residential facility may technically qualify as caregiving, it is almost assuredly not caring, since the aging person is not having her or his highly individual needs met in a personal and developmental fashion. Further, the perfunctory processing of families through an unfeeling welfare bureaucracy or the housing of persons with mental illness in a congregate institution may be statistically recorded as instances of caregiving, but caring will be in short supply. We argue that the ideal we should strive for individually and societally is to provide as many persons in need as possible—intimates and strangers alike—with caregiving that is truly caring.

Although these issues may appear to be abstract and more philosophical than practical, they have serious policy implications. As of 1990, we have more than 12 million people who live with a physical impairment and an additional 6.5 million who have one or more physical disabilities. Moreover, we can anticipate a profound increase in these numbers over the next fifty years given the projected "aging" of our population. When we include those persons with mental disability, the estimate is that 20 percent of our population—one in five—will need care for a problem of some significance.

Who provides this care? Who are the caregivers? Historically most have been family members, relatives, friends, and neighbors, disproportionately women. Today we refer to these as "informal caregivers" in the sense that they are not professionally trained for the caregiving task. The other source of caregivers is the professionals, those who provide care by virtue of their position and training. Often these two groups function independently, that is, *either* the informal *or* formal system is involved with a particular individual in need. At times, too infrequently, these two systems of caregiving come together in partnership. See Appendix A for our working definition of formal and informal caregivers.

What is the likelihood that these systems will be able to continue their caregiving? Furthermore, even if caregiving is provided, will it be caring, provided by caring people, whether they are from the informal or formal systems? Finally, what would happen if those in the informal system gave up the caregiving function?

Many people, without firm evidence, believe that the members of the informal support or caregiving system are typically unable or unwilling to be caregivers, or both. Often they reach these conclusions when they examine the changes occurring in America's families. Families today are different from earlier families in a number of ways. The proportion of married women who go out to work has risen dramatically; the traditional caregivers—the unemployed wife, daughter, or aunt—belong to a dwindling group, many of whom work outside the home or are otherwise unavailable as full-time caregivers. Additionally, the nature of dependency has changed (though not the overall ratio), with fewer children and more older persons. The increased rate of survival of severely handicapped children and the increased number of very old people, moreover, have also altered the dimensions and dynamics of care. The patterns of informal care have changed as well over the past two or three generations.

Only recently has our society begun to take note of the fact that the overwhelming majority of severely disabled persons are in the community and are being cared for by families and friends with varying degrees of support from public and voluntary agencies. This informal caregiving system has been instrumental in preventing or delaying many long-term admissions to institutions, thus reducing the heavy demand on our health and social welfare services. These families, often with the help of friends and neighbors, have provided what can only be described as a staggering amount of caregiving.

Many of these family members and friends, however, are undergoing considerable strain, and some question their physical or emotional ability to continue their caregiving functions. Many also wonder whether caregiving in the home and community serves the best interest of the care recipient's physical and social well-being and the best interest of the other family members.

If there is a growing trend in this direction, if caregivers are beginning to expect that society through its formal agencies and services should assume increased responsibility for the care of the disabled, and if this trend were to be expressed in greater demands on the service system, the social and economic ramifications would be significant. What would happen if even 5 to 10 percent of the caregivers who now look after their family members with disabilities asked the formal caregiving sector to assume this function?

The United States is currently faced with immense economic problems that are likely to continue for a number of years. Governments are emphasizing cutbacks in public expenditures, and state and local administrators feel pressured to limit their activities to those considered most pressing. An attitude of controlled retrenchment has replaced that of expansion, despite severe shortages in specific services that already exist, such as those that support caregivers. In periods of retrenchment, there is a rhetorical emphasis on supporting informal caregivers, while policy making and program development give priority to those persons with disabilities who do not have relatives, friends, and neighbors who are willing to provide or capable of providing such care. In relative terms, few resources are set aside to support the informal caregivers. The message, while implicit, is clear—wait until we can afford additional resources.

The purpose of this chapter is to define and make distinct the key concepts of *caring* and *caregiving* and discuss their relevance as a backdrop for developing an agenda for public policy. In the next chapter, we review diverse positions regarding actions that are appropriate and feasible for the informal system to take and those that are appropriate and realistic for formal systems to take when individuals are in need of substantial caregiving. We evaluate historical data in order to document changes in family types, structure, and functions in regard to families', friends', and relatives' ability to provide care to severely disabled people. With these data in mind, we discuss the currently vexing issues of diversity and equality. Following this, we identify in broad terms the types of formal support that would have benefit for informal caregivers. In later chapters we identify barriers to implementing a truly caring caregiving system. Finally, we offer a number of suggestions that we believe would help remedy the situation.

Caring and Cared-For Persons

We invite the reader to imagine the caring situation. You are a *caring person*. You are face to face with a person in need of care who summons the best in you, challenges you to relate to her or him as a *cared-for person*. Whether you are an *informal* caregiver (for example, a parent caring for a child, an adult child caring for a parent with Alzheimer's disease, a volunteer caring for a young child with Down's syndrome or for a dying person in a hospice) or a *formal* caregiver (such as a special education teacher caring for a student, a minister caring for a parishioner, a physician caring for a patient, or a therapist or social worker caring for a client), you are called upon to enter into a meaningful relationship.

When you care meaningfully, whether in a formal relationship or an informal one, two things can be said of you. First, in one way or another, your intentions and actions are focused on helping others to meet their fundamental human development needs—their need to grow; to respond to their life challenges in the context of a healthful and decent quality of life; to broaden their experiences; to develop and enlarge their realms of meaning; to actualize their potential; to be the best that they can be; to be, in Erik Erikson's (1967) term, "generative," a quality to be striven for throughout the whole course of human development (Browning 1973). Second, it can be said undeniably that you require a nurturing and supportive *community* to help meet the many challenges facing caregivers.

We define community here as a social grouping (for example, a nurturing family, a nourishing church, a supportive peer group or neighborhood, a compassionate school, a hospice) that promotes human development—one that *cares* for you. Not just any social grouping is a community in this sense. Indeed, one that hinders human development (for instance, a destructive dysfunctional family, a rigidly dogmatic church or a tyrannical cult, an alienated and hostile neighborhood, a school that menaces rather than teaches children, a sterile nursing home) would be an anticommunity. Its intentions and actions are not caring.

Like your own caring, true community enhances human development by increasing mutual aid and shared heritage among people and by not demeaning, dividing, or bestowing unwarranted advantage on them. It strengthens families, enables parents and other caregivers to do their jobs well, and respects the rights of all individuals. Anticommunities, on the other hand, are demeaning, divisive, and unfair. They weaken families, caregivers, and other individuals and thereby present obstacles to human development, even to the point of causing developmental setbacks and regression (Dokecki 1983; Hobbs et al. 1984; Moroney and Dokecki 1984).

Human development and community are two sides of the same coin— true community promotes human development; people who develop humanly seek to form or participate in community. Human development and community are *first principles,* fundamental ethical precepts: we *ought* to promote human development and community because they are fundamental purposes of human existence. And we *ought* to care because caring promotes human development and community.

The evidence for the importance and interrelationship of human development, community, and caring is voluminous. While this is not the place to review it, we assert that most schools of personality theory identify something like the sense of community and the process of human development as central (a) to our understanding of the person, (b) to whether the person experiences psychopathology and other developmental problems of living, and (c) to the degree to which the person experiences life as meaningful. Further, the theoretical and empirical literature on human development suggests that caring within supportive community environments is the sine qua non for human growth and development to occur. Finally, much of the Judeo-Christian, Western, and American ethical tradition identifies, either directly or indirectly, human development and community as central to the common good—that which is good for each of us in common and for our social life together in society. This is not to say that there are not different and valuable perspectives and understandings in both other Western traditions and non-Western traditions. In this time of increasing awareness and appreciation of multicultural ethical and social perspectives, the interrelationship of development, caring, and community as we have described it does, however, provide a useful framework within which we may pursue our analysis.

Caring encounters formidable challenges, for in many ways our society's structures do not support effective caring. Paradoxically, our society both increases the need for people to care and, at the same time, makes caregiving that is truly caring a difficult and challenging way of life. As with Sisyphus, caring entails rolling a very big rock up a very steep hill. We cannot claim to be fully human, however, unless we care. Caring is a challenge worthy of the best *in* us and the best *of* us.

What Is Caring?

Following Milton Mayeroff (1971),[1] we employ here a demanding "gold standard" for defining caring. Caring, says Mayeroff, is *not* several comfortable things you might at first think it to be. It is not merely wishing a person well, liking a person, or being interested in a person. It is not merely wanting to care. "My involvement was entirely voluntary. She is my mother, she is my responsibility, she is my blessing. It's a privilege to give the care."[2]

Parker (1981) distinguished between "caring" and "tending"; the former involves a concern about people; the latter describes the actual work of looking after those who cannot do for themselves. Graham (1983) amplifies Parker's framework and places great emphasis on "caring as a labor of love."

Leira (1994) offers a very helpful review of a number of different perspectives on this distinction. In citing one of her Scandinavian colleagues, she points out that Waerness has argued that affection and activity are closely related. "'Caring for' is embedded in 'caring about.' According to her [Waerness's] definition caregiving work demands not only a willingness to provide for the well-being of another person but also that the activity be performed with a positive, affectionate and loving attitude" (189).

Caring cannot be accomplished easily or quickly. For example, one caregiver surveyed by the Rosalynn Carter Institute said that caregiving for her loved one "caused severe financial stress; most other family members don't help; they are not around very much." Another caregiver said, "My life has been changed, and I feel helpless and filled with anger and frustration." "I have become hardened to problems. I have worked up a defense mechanism because you can only give so much without being totally empty," said a third caregiver.

Caring, therefore, as we have been suggesting, is not merely caregiving, as we have been using the term thus far. It entails many challenges. As we shall see, caregiving may or may not qualify as caring. Caring is a key standard we propose for caregivers, an ideal they should and, with appropriate support, could meet in their relationships with cared-for persons. What, then, is caring?

Caring Defined

Caring is helping a person grow—helping promote a person's human development. In referring to the person she cares for, a caregiver said that there is the "satisfaction of watching her grow and develop into a sound person." A formal caregiver said, "A female patient was sent to us in the fetal position, had been for so long. She had very bad bed sores and was uncommunicative. Now she can get to a sitting position in bed and the pressure sores are gone. She does make some desires and needs known by gestures and sounds now."

Caring potentially characterizes many kinds of relationships, such as those between parent and child, spouses, friends, teacher and student, therapist and client, physician and patient. Although there may be differences among these types of relationships, if they qualify as caring, they have a common pattern that goes beyond merely knowing and relating to a person on the surface; caring implies a personal level of experience. "Caregiving is more important than many other things in life," said one caregiver, and another said, "I've learned that it's really not just a job . . . but a commitment."

When you care, you enact a common pattern in which you experience another person both as *part* of you and *apart* from you and as needing to develop humanly. Devotion characterizes your response to the cared-for person, and her or his need gives direction to your caring actions. Interdependence—not independence, dependence, or codependence—best characterizes this part/apart relationship.

Your ability to foster the other person's human development affects your own well-being and human development. In other words, there is an interdependency between caregivers and care recipients. As several caregivers reported: "There is more understanding about yourself. There is personal fulfillment. It is good to know you are able to take care of someone." "My caregiving helps me; it changes the way you act." "I think I've gotten much stronger. I strengthened my values. It has enhanced my life definitely."

You feel needed by the other person to grow, to develop humanly, and you need the other's growth as a condition for your own growth and development. Thus, in caring, both the cared-for person and the person caring grow and develop. "I feel that she is happier and I am happy in the knowledge that she is well cared for," and "anytime you do for someone else, it improves you," said two caregivers. A third reported, "I believe that I can help a person at a crucial time in his life, and by making that person better, it makes me a better person. I believe in changes and I know I can make a difference in a person's life."

We must emphasize at this point, moreover, that certain boundary conditions—those involving persons in a comatose state, those with profound mental retardation or brain damage, those with advanced Alzheimer's disease, those in the final stages of AIDS or other terminal illnesses, and the like—can and should also be thought of in human development terms. The realm of human development is vast, and we should expand our understanding by seeing its reaches as extending to those who can be helped to experience such extreme conditions humanely and with dignity. We are calling for a logic and an outlook that, for example, would view dying as the final stage of human development; therefore, a hospice would be considered to be an excellent instance of caring.

The often spoken reason for entering a caregiving profession is that it will help the professional grow and find meaning. This may be problematic. If you choose to care for the other person because you want to grow—if you selfishly put your own needs before those of the other—you may not only be failing to care but may also be using the other as a means to your own ends, treating the other as an object to be used for your own purposes. In many professional ethical codes, this constitutes a problematic dual relationship, an abuse of power, which is often the basis for breaches of ethics. Caring enables you to grow, *if* you intend your caring actions to benefit the person cared for. This seems paradoxical, but it is essential to understanding caring's truly interdependent nature. Said one caregiver, "My ideas have changed from wanting to be a person people depend upon to be a person that encourages independence. I don't want my clients to need me in every aspect of their lives, just know if they do need me, I'm available." In a particularly vivid way, another caregiver said:

> The longer I practice, the more responsibility I put on the patient. I put myself out of a job. I want the client to find the answer in themselves. I use the analogy of training wheels. The client should rely on me, only for awhile, until he learns to ride on his own. He may wobble, he may fall down, but he should have the strength within himself to pick up and go on. When you first come out of school, you want to take everyone under your wing. This is not in the client's best interest.

Unfortunately, many instances of caregiving result in exploitative, dependency-inducing, and codependent forms of relationship and thereby do not meet the standard of caring we develop here. Moreover, not only those cared for may suffer exploitation. When society coerces people into providing care, they experience a form of exploitation, as when women assume the caregiving role because of the social pressure engendered by the traditional stereotype that women are the obvious and "natural" ones for caregiving and are expected to do so whether they want to or not.

As a caring person, says Mayeroff, you help others grow—and you in turn grow—through a process of enabling them (a) to care for other persons beyond themselves, (b) to identify or create their own domains of caring, (c) to care for themselves, and (d) to take responsibility for their own lives. "You have to let patients take responsibility for themselves. You're really here to give them another perspective on their lives," said one caregiver.

In a sense, the caregiver should have dual goals: the growth of the care recipient and the growth of self. These features of the caring process, of course, are conditional on the status of the cared-for person. In the boundary conditions already mentioned (coma, profound mental retardation or brain damage, advanced Alzheimer's disease, the final stages of AIDS or other terminal illnesses, and the like), to the extent possible you help these persons grow, keeping in mind that humane care in pursuit of living and dying with dignity is the goal of those seeking to enhance human development.

Growing, for its part, says Mayeroff, entails *learning,* understood not as the accumulation of facts and skills but as enlarging one's scope of understanding by increasing one's experiences and integrating them into one's meaning system. Growing also entails *becoming self-determining*—breaking away from slavish conformity, choosing one's values, making one's own decisions, and taking responsibility for them. Moreover, learning and becoming self-determining occur within relationships, not in social isolation. Said one caregiver, "We want to help and we do that by our relationship. How we reach the patient is based on the relationship we have. This determines what they can use. You can go to someone, but if you can't touch them, then they can't use your help."

Caring, as we have been developing the concept, entails a caring and a cared-for person enhancing each other's human development, in effect, helping each other to grow, to become capable of meeting life's challenges in an ethical and meaningful manner. Usually, however, there are "dry spells" and frustrations when growth is elusive, sometimes caused by society's failure to respect the personhood of all, especially minority group members and women. The caregiver often gets stuck in this duality of relationships and needs the introduction of a third party—for example, a support group—to unbalance things. Although we have been suggesting that where there is no development there is no caring—a truly demanding standard—the pattern of your actions over time, not every particular action, should produce development if you are really caring. A pervasive and general failure to influence development, however, should be a signal that societal conditions should be addressed or that you should revise or expand your understanding of the cared-for person. This demand for influencing development—enhancing the personhood of the one being cared for—is a major reason that caring is so challenging.

The Ingredients of Caring

What must the caring person be like? And what must the caring person do? Mayeroff has much to teach about the ingredients of caring. These ingredients do not presume or necessitate a hierarchical structure or position of power out of which the caring person cares and the cared-for person is a passive recipient of care. Let us, then, follow his reasoning and examine caring's eight basic elements: knowing, alternating rhythms, patience, honesty, trust, humility, hope, and courage.

Although caring may seem to reside mostly in emotional or attitudinal domains, perhaps its most important ingredient, says Mayeroff, is *knowing*, itself a process with integrated emotional, attitudinal, and intellectual aspects. In a caring relationship, knowing necessarily occurs in a variety of ways and at various levels. The one who cares knows *who* the cared-for person is—his or her needs, his or her strengths, his or her weaknesses. The one who cares also knows his or her own needs, strengths, and weaknesses. The caring person knows the most appropriate ways of responding to the other's needs—including the most appropriate and valid techniques—in order to influence growth. Said one caregiver:

> Ten years ago when I worked with crippled children, a woman gave birth to a little girl with many congenital defects—the mother totally rejected the baby but the father was devoted to it. I took this family on and went everyday to see that the baby was fed and taken care of. The mother wouldn't even look at it, no matter what I said or did. One day I pretended I was ill and suddenly had to dash to the bathroom. I literally plunged the baby into the mother's arms.

I waited in the bathroom for a long while. When I came out, the mother was sitting on the sofa—cooing at the baby. I came back that evening when the father came home—when he saw his wife holding the baby, it was a wonderful experience. I'm still very close to the family—the girl grew up to be a wonderful young woman.

This instance of knowing may not be in the textbooks, but it demonstrates that caring requires immediate, intimate, and practical knowledge in order to enhance human development. Mayeroff's second ingredient of caring is *alternating rhythms.* Caring is not a linear process. Its rhythms are many and varied. They include moving back and forth between doing, experiencing, and evaluating the results of your doing. Sometimes even doing nothing is the appropriate way to care. There is also the need to alternate between a broad and a narrow perspective on the person being cared for, on yourself, on your caring actions, and on the environment surrounding the caring relationship. At times the total picture affords you the best option for providing care, and at other times a narrower view is more productive. Alternating your perspective and your actions helps to keep you in rhythmic connection with the changing needs of the cared-for person and with her responses to your actions and the world around her.

Since you ground caring in the uniqueness of the persons cared for, you manifest that ingredient of caring called *patience.* Patience means allowing cared-for persons to grow in their own time. Said one caregiver:

> It's the rare occasion when you get some kind of immediate response. Often you don't know what you said to make a difference someone will come back and say, "What you said last week really made me think, I feel so much better." You may not remember saying the one thing that helped the most. I'm more realistic. Caregivers can't change the world. The most powerful impact we can have is to be in touch with ourselves—be a model for our patients. I've become more empathetic, more accepting of people for who they are and where they are. I'm more patient now.

Patience also means that there are times to act and times to wait. Waitful caring, however, is not passive but actively chosen because that is what the caring moment requires. You also are patient in tolerating confusion. Someone once facetiously defined genius as the patience to delay making a decision in a confusing situation until the last possible moment before chaos sets in. Finally, you are patient with yourself in giving yourself time to master the challenges of caring.

Another ingredient of a caring person is *honesty*. As a caring person, you are honest with yourself and with the cared-for person. You view people as they are, not in a romanticized or glorified fashion. "Be candid and honest, don't just tell what they want to hear," said one caregiver. But not only do you not lie; you also actively embody the truth by living authentically and "ringing true." This is a matter of being the self you truly are as a caring person and not hiding behind facades, including techniques, defenses, titles, or credentials. You are willing to admit mistakes and take steps to correct them. Said another formal caregiver, "Professionals need to be real honest that they don't have the answers—that life is an experience that we will walk together and share. Through sharing, answers will come."

As a caring person, says Mayeroff, you establish and manifest the ingredient of *trust*. You trust your own caring capacity and the cared-for person's capacity to change. Trust here implies your willingness to take risks, to enter unknown realms as the caring situation demands it. In addition, you are, in effect, a trustworthy trustee—you can be trusted not to abuse power and not to take advantage of your caring position. Entailed here is sharing responsibility with cared-for persons so they may maintain, or come to gain, power over their lives. As one caregiver put it:

> As professionals, we have a tendency to feel a bit superior—we don't give the client and family sufficient credit to tell us what they need. We need to let them voice their needs, in their own terms. We need to provide services in a caring, kind manner and then we need to get out, we must know when not to interfere. Empower the patient. Everyone should encircle the patient, working to empower the patient to do what needs to be done.

Humility as an ingredient of true caring is multifaceted. It entails your willingness to admit what you don't know and to learn more about the caring process and the persons involved in it, including yourself. As one caregiver, a physician, put it:

> Often the families have the knowledge of the patient and the patient's desires, and the professional must listen to the family. The professional does have the knowledge education and training brings, but often we see, or sometimes fail to see, the understanding and sensitivities that family members bring to their caring for the patient. There are times when the professional must support the family. They must recognize when this need arises. Doctors should listen to the patient, the family. Doctors need to know more about all

the resources available. They can often learn from the lay caregiver. They must remain receptive.

Humility also means, as we have seen, not caring primarily to meet your own needs and not abusing your power. It means recognizing your limitations, but it doesn't rule out your taking pride in caring well done—caregiving that results in human development. True humility must be distinguished from the situation in which people are coerced into performing caregiving roles, as with many women and members of disadvantaged groups, and thus feel powerless, not because they are humble about their power but because they are victims of the power of others and are themselves in need of empowerment.

The virtue of *hope* is one of caring's central ingredients. Hope means not being presumptuous or cocky about what you can accomplish. But it also means you are not despairing about your ability to care meaningfully and effectively in challenging and frustrating circumstances. Hope as an ingredient of caring, moreover, entails action, not passive waiting. Hope is the expectation that the future is full of possibilities to be actualized through your caring actions and the actions of the cared-for person, although with many women and members of minority groups, society interferes with their feeling hopeful in the difficult and stressful circumstances they are forced to occupy.

The last ingredient of caring that we shall consider is the virtue of *courage.* Courage relates to trust: it entails your willingness to enter unknown realms. Courage here is not foolhardiness; rather, it is founded on the wisdom gained from past experience, the accurate understanding of the present, and the informed expectation of future possibilities.

Caring, Difference, and Justice

In this chapter, we have been suggesting that caring is a defining aspect of being human. A crucially important dimension of the human condition that affects caring is human diversity—persons differ from one another in a great many ways. These differences include age, gender, culture, race, ethnicity, nationality, socioeconomic status, religion, and sexual preference. We hotly debate the implications of these differences. They engender anxiety, defensiveness, and, in the extreme, fear. Our position in this book is that we should not only endure and "deal with" human diversity but also value and celebrate it.

Caring Requires Diversity

Diversity challenges us to grow and is an occasion for creativity and social insight. It is stitched into the fabric of caring relationships but often, unfortunately, in problematic ways. As we shall discuss in the next chapter, (a) women, not men, inordinately provide the care in our society; (b) adults care for the very young and the very old, often in the face of obstacles and without adequate support; (c) socioeconomically disadvantaged persons and members of minority groups often need more care but find it to be inaccessible. In other words, diversity as a social good is often the source of injustice and exploitation in the realm of caring as in the rest of society: certain groups take advantage of the vulnerabilities of the "different ones," and we have ageism, sexism, racism, economic exploitation, religious prejudice, and other forms of intolerance, lack of charity, and close-mindedness—all of which undermine the human community.

Caring Requires Justice

Justice demands that equality be the core value guiding society's response to human differences in the provision of care. Rather than serving as the basis for injustice, diversity calls us to recognize the common needs and common risks experienced by all people and to transcend characteristics that make us distinct. This is a traditional American position: all human beings are created equal and must be accorded the status of a person, that is, we must (a) be accorded necessary care and thereby experience human development and a sense of community, (b) be responsible for caring for others, and (c) be supported in caring by appropriate societal institutions and public policies.

Caring Requires Equality

Equality in pursuit of caring is difficult to achieve in the postmodern world. Vested political, economic, and social interests and long-standing prejudices interfere. We have typically relied on governmental interventions to help rectify injustice. This form of societal intervention will continue to be necessary to recognize the personhood of all in the provision of necessary care. Democracy in the modern era has tried, at least theoretically, to structure institutions so that we consult the "bottom up" when the "top down" enacts decisions. This consultation, however, has often been inadequate and merely procedural. Whatever the future holds in store, if caring is to become a priority, participatory decision making must be fostered.

Caring Requires Participatory Decision Making

The interplay of diversity, justice, equality, and participatory decision making creates challenging and complicated social relations at this time in U.S. history. The undeniable fact of human differences is as fundamental to the phenomenon of caring as any other single dimension of social life. To foster caring requires, in short, paying attention to the pluralism in American society.

"Difference" is a focus of much discussion in many areas, including ethnic and women's studies. Often these discussions seek to clarify the relationship between human similarities and differences. When we speak glibly of these similarities as universals within which we collapse all differences and diversity, we may overlook particular and concrete situations. In failing to attend to the particular and the concrete, we may severely restrict and limit our ability to care. On the other hand, we may equally speak too glibly of human differences in ways that seem to deny all human similarities, in ways that are contentious and socially divisive. In either case, we often end up talking at or past one another rather than engaging in *conversations of mutuality*—conversations through which we come to learn more competent and caring ways of caregiving. Extreme emphasis either on similarities/universals or on differences/diversity prevents the kind of intimately shared knowing between persons that encourages the mutual relationships required in caring.

Human need—in the many forms and degrees encountered by professional and informal caregivers—is of fundamental concern. Whatever policy and service delivery changes may be in the offing, caregivers must be encouraged to identify those services that they believe to be important to their ability to continue providing care. "Top-down" service philosophies and policies that fail to encourage such valid needs assessment will fall far short of caring.

A question vital to similarity-difference discussions is similar to one often posed in discussions regarding change: Who stands to gain and lose when changes occur? The assumption that all persons have similar needs often guides our theorizing and policy making. This assumption tends to maintain the status quo of the existing society and service system. If we seek to hear the voices of the "different ones," then we must make changes (in theory, in policy, in method, in service delivery, and the like)—changes that challenge the norm, the expected. These changes caused by paying attention to diversity may threaten service system administrators and professionals, who may perceive that they are losing some of their discretion and power. They may believe that spending more time listening and using participatory decision making is inefficient, even counterproductive. Yet, without providing the time, space, and opportunity for hearing from the caregivers and care recipients, will the services we develop be the services that will make a difference in their lives? Somehow, we must move away from this societally conditioned win-lose framework toward one where we view caring that addresses diversity as a win-win proposition—win-win because caregivers are pleased to actualize their potential through caring, and those in need of care in fact receive care.

The topic of human differences often remains unaddressed or underaddressed, and diversity-related changes are often resisted or minimized. These concerns involve assumptions important to any discussion of care and caregiving. Critical attention to the significance of both difference and similarity in caregiving philosophy, policy, method, and practice reveals complexities at every level, complexities that already exist, not ones created by the greater recognition. The need is for clear and accurate needs assessment. This process requires a willingness, and appropriate methods, for engaging in mutuality and listening as caregivers seek to hear the many different voices of race, ethnicity, age, gender, sexual orientation, physical ability, income, and the like, in caring conversations.

These concerns regarding similarities and differences in caregiving are not only theoretical but also practical and political in nature. "Who stands to gain and lose?" or "What is gained or lost?" or "Which questions do we ask or not ask, and why?" are caring questions. They need to be addressed in order to better understand how we are currently assessing and addressing caregiving needs.

This focus on difference and similarity is vital in developing more responsive approaches in caregiving policies, systems, methods, and practices. It may help us hear the voices—expressing values, experiences, concerns, understandings—of the many different kinds of caregivers and persons in need of care involved in potentially caring relationships. A diversity of caregiving methods is not enough, however, especially when those methods derive from systems imposed from above with only minimal participation from the caregivers and receivers. More fundamental, respectful, mutually engaged learning from human differences—differences that already exist and pervade daily caregiving realities—is one important way of increasing care in caregiving.

These aspects of caring and caregiving need to be examined more closely in the context of present-day life. How realistic is such a formulation? What are the forces that facilitate or hinder caring? Many societal and cultural factors challenge the caring way of life in our contemporary world, matters we begin to explore in the next chapter.

2০ Caregiving:
Facts, Trends, Realities

THERE ARE numerous current views on caregiving; some represent facts, and others are myths. Current conventional wisdom reflects an apparent consensus that the family as an institution has changed over time in structure, form, and activity patterns, with the most significant changes having occurred in the last fifty or sixty years. Many who are central to public discourse believe that, because of these changes, people today are less willing to carry out certain functions for which families have historically assumed responsibility, especially caregiving to disabled or needful members.

Yet our nation's position on the family has not been consistent over time. For the past sixty or so years, we have shifted our beliefs and public policies, sometimes in drastic and contradictory ways. At least two major paradigms have emerged over this period—each with a different perspective on the appropriate role families assume in meeting the needs of their members (Moroney 1991).

Our primary approach to families and caregiving from approximately the 1930s until the 1970s encompassed several major principles. Because of the depression and its attendant massive unemployment and related problems, we were forced to accept the fact that the typically American perspective of "rugged individualism" and minimal government involvement in private and family matters was no longer pragmatic. Private efforts were clearly inadequate in meeting the growing needs experienced by millions of depression-era Americans. When individuals, families, and private organizations on their own could not entirely care for persons in need, public intervention was called for, and government became ever more involved in meeting human needs. This belief generated programs ranging from public education to social insurance to national health insurance.

An important corollary to this type of intervention was a serious questioning of earlier beliefs about human nature and about those who sought or received assistance.

> We began to believe that we could enhance family and community life if we gave caregivers relief from onerous caregiving tasks. From this belief emerged policies establishing programs such as homemaker/home care services, respite care, information and referral, and even financial support.
>
> We also came to believe that professionals were essential to providing effective services since they were grounded in the theory and practice of effective intervention and they understood the interdependency of the formal and informal caregiving system.

In sum, for much of the middle years of this century, society (as expressed in public policy) assumed that most people recognized their natural obligation to care for one another but understood that caregiving individuals and their families were experiencing heightened and often unbearable stress resulting from rapid economic and social changes. We acknowledged that continuing shifts in our economic system produced risks and consequences that negatively affected the quality of individual and family life, thus requiring society, through public agencies, to create a safety net.

In the 1970s, an older paradigm began to reemerge, one with its roots in the Poor Law of the nineteenth century. This older view in new garb, increasingly voiced until today, arose in part because of the economic crises brought on by rising inflation and oil-related problems, which brought into question the continuing funding of many social programs. Growing lack of trust in government attendant on the Vietnam War and the Watergate scandal exacerbated these economic difficulties, leading to an emerging perspective on families that incorporated several beliefs:

> We began to believe that government efforts to improve the quality of life of individuals and families are often not only undesirable but harmful. This is a variation of the sometimes voiced argument that governmental intervention weakens families by creating dependency.
>
> We believed that we should not relieve people of traditional caregiving tasks since they often see public intervention as interference, interpretable by many caregivers as a lack of trust in their ability to care.
>
> We believed that we should decentralize decision making for those in need because of our assumption that the greater the distance between decision

making authority and those in need the less is the sensitivity and conscientiousness of the decision maker.

We began to believe that professionals are self-serving and intentionally create dependency to meet their own needs.

In sum, emerging national beliefs suggest in this "newer" paradigm that too much has already been done for families, that the formal caregiving system is overdeveloped, that families have been weakened, and that they need to reassume many of their traditional caregiving tasks—even in instances where they may not want to do so. We are critical of proactive government and policies that are universal in coverage. Under this newer paradigm—representing principles of staunch individualism and utilitarianism—government assumes a reactive stance, intervening only in instances of clearly defined pathology.

Although it seemed there might be an interest in returning to the earlier activist government paradigm in the public arena over the past few years (for example, President Clinton's aborted national health plan proposal, with its provisions for universal coverage), the newer minimalist government paradigm continues to be very strong. Recent concerns about the national budget deficit and the attendant fear of the size and scope of government have strengthened it. Actually, we seem to vacillate in our beliefs about families, holding contradictory views about their capacities and intentions and the degree to which government should be active. One fundamental theme is the belief that most people, most of the time, can take care of their own needs and that only a few people—a residual—fall by the wayside and need help from the more formal and impersonal institutions beyond their immediate circle. This *residual approach* carries an assumption that people who seek help from formal sources do so, at least partially, because of personal or family deficits and pathology.

The fact that the residual group has become a large group challenges the residual assumption: a steadily growing number of individuals and families have left the mainstream of self-sufficiency. Yet social policy still tends to provide services based on deficits, which assumes that most people can and should be self-sufficient. Social policy, moreover, identifies recipients of aid on the basis of poverty. A common assumption is that those with greater means do not need support of any kind from the formal system or, if they do, they can pay for it. These perspectives derive from historically deeply held notions about the family as the basic unit of community life. As Demos (1983) suggests:

> Families [in the eighteenth and nineteenth centuries] were the building blocks from which all larger units of social organizations could be fashioned. A family was itself a little society. . . . The family performed a multitude of functions, both for the individual and for the aggregate to which it belonged. Thus, most of what children received by way of formal education was centered around the home hearth; likewise their training in particular vocations, in religious worship, and in what we would call good citizenship. Illness was also a matter of home care. (164)

Communities then were settings in which families interacted with other families for mutual support. The classic example is that of a barn raising—where the total community came together to build a home or barn for a family in need. People willingly gave of their time and resources to help others with the understanding that if they ever needed assistance it would be available.

This ideal of the rural family, real or not, is the family prototype around which we have built much of our public policy. Consistent with the belief that government intervention in the economy should be minimal and undertaken only after clear imperfections in specific markets, we also believe that government should not interfere with family life. Intervention should be limited to those instances in which family functioning is clearly impaired so that we may help the residual few who cannot help themselves. Helping others can be dangerous, since they might become weakened because we have intervened (Moroney 1991).

The belief is that family life is and should be a private matter. Many view the family as a haven in the harsh economic world, and, therefore, believe government should not interfere in its internal affairs. Further, the family is perceived to be a fragile institution, one that is "besieged" and must be protected (Lasch 1978). This approach supports the notion of intervention in family life only when necessary. In this outlook, it is not that we lack interest in all families, nor do we deny that all families could use supportive services. The concern is a fundamental one: that intervention might result in families giving up their responsibilities—responsibilities they would or should prefer to keep. Instead of helping families remain strong caregiving units, what we call support might weaken the family.

Help becomes interference. Therefore, the appropriate role for the formal caregiving system is to become involved only when there is clear evidence of the informal caregiving system's inability to function adequately. By waiting until the family declares its inability to care for a disabled member, for example, the formal system can be sure that its involvement is necessary. Since there is such a fine line between intervention and interference in this outlook, caution is the preferred course.

This line of argument is usually supported with the assertion that families have deteriorated—an assertion based on social indicators (for example, rates of out-of-wedlock pregnancy, divorce, family violence, delinquency, adolescent pregnancies, and chronic economic dependency). The resultant list of weak family types, then, includes single-parent and "broken" families, families in which parents abuse themselves or their children, families whose adolescents behave in sexually or violently disruptive ways, families on public welfare, and the like. The argument inevitably leads to proposals to rehabilitate or, at times, reconstitute these families, to make them more like strong families—families that care for their own members with little outside help.

An example of this position is the argument offered by a major spokesperson associated with the "profamily" movement in this country.

> Families are strong when they have a function to perform, and when the government takes over the functions of the family, then as sure as night follows day, families are going to disintegrate and fall apart, because they have no reason to exist. . . . Today we have well intentioned causes saying that we will provide your food and we'll take care of your health, and we'll provide you with everything you really need, and then you can be a strong family. It doesn't work that way. We have seen the results of that kind of misguided policy. Families are strong when they have a job to do. (Marshner 1981, 63)

This position has currency beyond the boundaries of this country. For example, a decade earlier, Sir Keith Joseph, a leader of England's Conservative Party and an adviser to Margaret Thatcher, suggested:

> [The family and civilized values] are the foundation on which the nation is built; they are being undermined. If we cannot restore them to health, our nation can be utterly ruined, whatever economic policies we might try to follow. . . . The socialist would try to take away from the family and its members the responsibilities which gives it cohesion. Parents are being divested of their

duty to provide for their family economically, of their responsibility for education, health and upbringing, morality, advice and guidance, of saving for old age, for housing. When you take responsibility away from people you make them irresponsible. (Joseph 1974, 5)

What we see, then, is a widespread belief that not only are people less willing to provide care, or less capable of doing so, to family members or disabled persons outside their immediate family, but the cause is the evolution and expansion of the current health and social welfare system. Government efforts, since the depression, to improve the quality of life for families and individuals are viewed as both undesirable and harmful in that they invariably weaken people and create dependency. When the formal system (both the governmental and voluntary sectors) provides more and more services, families begin to feel that they are neither capable nor expected to continue their traditional responsibilities. Finally, it is argued that families should not be relieved of their caregiving responsibilities unless we are prepared to see them transfer more and more of them to the formal system.

These are not new fears. They existed in various forms prior to the depression, prior to the advent of the modern welfare state. Sorokin (1946) raised the same warnings in the early 1920s when he spoke of the crisis then facing Western society—a crisis that was, in his opinion, destroying the fundamental institutions in society. While he saw that this deterioration affected all social institutions, his comments related to the family are most germane:

> The Family is virtually non-existent nowadays. In contradistinction to the medieval family or even that of a century ago. As it has become more and more contractual, the family of the last few decades has grown even more unstable, until it has reached the point of actual disintegration. . . . The result is . . . an increasing number of young people without moral integrity, strength of character, a sense of social duty or spontaneous altruism, . . . who swell the ranks of irresponsible persons. (181)

These positions, all from the twentieth century, are still only a partial picture. If we look back further still, a considerable amount of evidence was presented to England's Royal Commission on the Poor Laws concluding that virtually the same crisis described by Sorokin and our more recent examples existed in that country since the beginning of the seventeenth century. The testimony had a familiar ring concerning "the disinclination of relatives to assist one another." It reported,

> It appears from the whole evidence that the clause of the 43rd Eliz (enacted in 1601) which directs the parents and children of the impotent to be assessed for their support, is very seldom enforced. In any ordinary state of society, we much doubt the wisdom of such an enactment. The duty of supporting parents and children in old age or infirmity is so strongly enforced by ones natural feelings, that it is well performed even among savages and almost always in a society deserving the name of civilized. We believe we are the only country in which it is neglected. (Report of the Poor Law Commission of 1832, 43)

But England was not the only country experiencing the "deterioration of the family" (43).

The American colonies adopted the same Elizabethan Poor Law including the family responsibility clause. By 1836, all states on the Atlantic seaboard, with the exception of New York, expanded this clause to include the legal responsibility of grandchildren to care for their grandparents (Coll 1973, 21).

What conclusions can be drawn from this retracing of the past? One is that people in each successive generation, when confronted with some crisis, invariably looked to the family as it then existed, disliked what they saw, and suggested that the crisis could only be averted if the family became more like the family they thought existed in the past. Another is that each generation might have held up too high an ideal.

While the conclusions have been similar over the centuries, the same cannot be said for the perceived cause. Some saw the reasons as spiritual (attributable to the presence or absence of religion), others as biological (a regression toward the mean resulting in the inevitable deterioration of the human genetic stock) or physical (sun spots or climactic shifts). The most recurring argument sees the cause in social-political-economic terms, and the dominant economic system, whether capitalism or socialism, has received its share of the blame.

The present concern about family well-being and capability, then, is not unique to our time. As a theme it can be found in generations preceding the twentieth century. Although it might be an interesting exercise to trace this theme back even further than the seventeenth century, to attempt to find that period when a generation would state that the family was better off than families of previous generations, one may assume that, once the apple was eaten and the gates of Paradise closed, no such claim would have been made. Large numbers of people over the ages have believed that their generation's families are weaker than those of earlier generations, and this belief disturbs them. The recent wave of nostalgia about life in the past and family life in particular is a good example of this. The media (theater, literature, television) tend to glorify and romanticize the past: it was a better time to have lived; life was less complex; and appropriate values were respected. Since many in this generation have reached the same conclusion, we must ask whether they are speaking of a past they knew, one they imagine, or a past they need to believe existed even if it did not. This pattern has been labeled "the world we have lost syndrome" (Laslett 1976).

Caregiving: Demographic Realities

We generally believe that people in the past were more caring and more responsible than people are today. We hear complaints that aged parents are shunted off to nursing homes or retirement homes by their adult children and that children and adults with severe disabilities are sent to institutions. Research data, as incomplete as they are, do not support these claims, suggesting, rather, that most family members in the past did not face this institutionalization decision, that fewer people survived to old age, and that most people who were born with a severe disability died very young.

It has been estimated that as many as 2.5 percent of the adult population are physically disabled. Disability, of course, can be defined in a number of ways, and various estimates of prevalence are derived depending on the definition used. For our purposes, a functional definition of disability would seem more appropriate than a diagnostic one in order to determine how much caregiving occurs and what it entails (Moroney 1986).

More than 910,000 Americans may be classified functionally as *very severely disabled.* This grouping includes those who are unable to understand questions or give rational answers because of cognitive impairment or senility; those who are permanently bedridden; those who are confined to a chair, unable to get in or out without assistance, and unable to feed themselves; and those who are doubly incontinent or cannot be left alone

TABLE 2.1. Elderly Population, 1900–2000

Year	Total U.S. Population	Ages 65–74	Ages 75–84	Over 84	%>64
1900	76,094,000	2,337,000	661,000	122,000	4.1
2000	265,000,000	17,230,000	10,505,000	3,254,000	11.9
% Increase	248%	637%	1,489%	2,567%	

Source: Adapted from U.S. Bureau of the Census, "Demographic Aspects of Aging and the Older Population in the United States," Current Population Reports Special Studies Series P-23 (Washington, D.C.: GPO, 1989).

because they might harm themselves. An additional 2,179,000 are *severely disabled.* These include persons who experience difficulty doing every- thing or find most things difficult and some things impossible to do. The *appreciably disabled,* approximately 3,509,000 adults, can do a fair amount for themselves but have difficulty with some activities and need assistance to carry them out.

Disability is not evenly distributed across age groups. Sixty-four per- cent of all disabled persons are elderly; 72 percent of these are very severely disabled. The elderly over seventy-four years of age are 2.5 times more likely to be very severely disabled than are those between sixty-five and seventy-four years of age.

Since 1900, the elderly population has increased at a rate far greater than that of the general population as life expectancy has increased from approximately thirty-five years at the beginning of the nineteenth century, to forty-nine years at the turn of the twentieth century, to seventy-six years today. By the year 2000, fourteen million persons will be over seventy-four years of age, and one in ten—more than three million people—will be eighty years of age or older.

Data on physically disabled children and youth are more difficult to find. Riley and Nagi (1980) state that 2 per 1,000 persons under the age of seventeen are disabled. This seems to be reasonable given the estimate of 1.9 per 1,000 for those aged sixteen to twenty-nine (Moroney 1986).

Taking the rates of 2 per 1,000 under seventeen years of age, we can es- timate that the total physically disabled population in 2000 will be more than 6.5 million children and adults. This significant number of people make up a population that is at risk and one that uses or needs a high volume of health and social services. This group also makes heavy demands upon caregivers, who, by virtue of their caregiving roles, must live differently from most people and face stressors not shared by the rest of the population.

In addition, Manderscheid and Sonnerschein (1992) have estimated that there are some four to five million persons with chronic mental disability over the age of eighteen and approximately half a million children under the age of eighteen with serious emotional disability. These are people who experience limitations in work, school, personal care, social functioning, and coping with the stresses associated with daily living. Not all people, however, are as likely to experience mental disabilities. Those living in poverty are 2.5 times more likely to have problems in this area; and those with less than a high school education are twice as likely.

Given these data, we can estimate that more than eleven million children and adults are either physically or mentally disabled and need supportive services. Is today's informal caregiving system less willing or less able to provide care than were caregivers one hundred years ago? The data suggest some answers. Clearly, the number of individuals needing care was much lower at the turn of the twentieth century and has grown significantly during the past one hundred years. It will continue to grow given increased life expectancy and more effective medical intervention for disabled infants and children.

It is almost impossible to predict beyond the year 2000. The prevalence of Alzheimer's disease will undoubtedly increase given the aging of the population. Moreover, the incidence of AIDS and new viral diseases is increasing at an extremely high rate. These two conditions alone will place tremendous demands on those who provide care—both formal and informal caregivers.

Also relevant to the question of informal caregivers' willingness and ability to provide care is the rate of institutionalization. How many persons live in institutions? Are the numbers increasing?

Since 1950, slightly more than 1 percent of the population has been institutionalized (excluding correctional facilities and the military) at any one time. Although there have been shifts in the rates of institutionalization within types of facilities (for example, many of the elderly were moved from mental hospitals to nursing homes following the introduction of Medicaid in 1965), the overall rate has remained remarkably constant.

TABLE 2.2. Infant Mortality Rates, 1920–1990
(per 1,000 live births)

1920	85.8
1940	47.0
1960	26.0
1970	26.0
1980	12.6
1990	10.0

Sources: U.S. Bureau of the Census, *Historical Statistics of the United States: From Colonial Times to 1957* (Washington, D.C.: GPO, 1960), 23–25; U.S. Bureau of the Census, *Census of Population: Current Population Reports, Household and Family Characteristics,* Series P-20, Number 467 (Washington, D.C.: GPO, 1992); National Center for Health Statistics, *Monthly Vital Statistics Report* (Washington, D.C.: GPO, 1992).

The institutionalization rate has dropped, however, for each grouping below the age of seventy, with the largest decrease seen for those under fifteen years of age. It is clear that institutionalization is not the norm; in all age groupings, rates of institutionalization are significantly lower than disability rates. Most handicapped persons, regardless of age, are living in the community (for instance, in community facilities such as shelters or small group homes; alone in their own homes; and in the homes of their parents, their adult children, or their siblings).

Despite these data, recent surveys of values and beliefs associated with family life, marriage, personal expectations, and roles of adults would seem to work against the provision of home-based care. Such care is demanding and disruptive, and it requires family members, especially adult women, to make major life adjustments. And yet, most families apparently choose to provide care for their own, often for long periods of time, though they may also call upon many adjunct sources of care such as neighbors, friends, and volunteers. In fact, Nottingham et al. (1993) found that 97 percent of formal caregivers and 88 percent of informal caregivers reported caregiving to be personally rewarding. These results suggest that caregiving, especially for informal caregivers, is simultaneously rewarding and burdensome.

While not all caregivers experience the same level of stress, nor are they confronted with identical stressors, all who provide care are at risk. Still, there are significant commonalities in the types of strain they encounter. These pressures often include the additional financial costs associated with the disability (Aldrich et al. 1971; Baldwin 1985; Joshi 1987; Martin and White 1988; Sultz et al. 1972), stigma, time consumed in personal care (feeding, washing, dressing) (Newman 1976; Dunlap 1976), difficulties with physical management (lifting, ambulation), decline in the physical well-being of the caregiver (Sainsbury and Grad de Alarcon 1971; Hewett 1972), interruption of sleep, social isolation (Gottlieb 1975), limitations in recreational activities (Justice, Bradley, and O'Connor 1971; Parker 1992; Twigg and Atkin 1993), and management of behavioral problems (Bayley 1973). Some caregivers also face stressors associated with balancing home and work schedules and balancing the needs of other family members with the needs of the member with disabilities (Bone, Spain, and Martin 1972; Farber 1975; Wilkin 1979; Glendinning 1983). For a comprehensive and up-to-date review of this literature, see Twigg (1992).

Characteristics of the American Family

While neighbors, friends, and volunteers carry some of the burden of the informal caregiving system and are themselves subject to special stress and strain, it is the family that has traditionally provided what Bayley (1973) has referred to as "the mundane slog of caring" (48)—the continuous day-to-day concern and attentiveness required by persons with disabilities. Are today's families effective caregivers? If so, will they be able to continue to be so in the future?

Families today differ significantly from those of the nineteenth century, and a number of the differences potentially affect their capability and willingness to care for their dependent members. Families have become smaller; they have more older and dependent members, reflecting the shifting composition of the population at large; and the number of single-parent families has increased sharply. Like families throughout history, however, they tend to look to their female members as primary care-givers—raising questions of justice—even though women have entered the workforce in significant numbers and their earnings account for an important part of the average family's total income. These and other re-lated facts suggest that the structure and means of family caregiving are undergoing profound change. Although it is not correct to say that today's

TABLE 2.3. Family Size, 1930–1990 (in Percentages)

# Persons	1930	1940	1950	1980	1990
2	26.1	29.3	32.8	39.9	40.8
3	22.5	24.2	25.2	23.0	23.9
4	18.8	19.3	19.8	20.6	21.1
5	12.8	11.7	11.1	9.7	9.1
6	8.1	6.8	5.6	3.2	3.2
7	11.7	8.7	5.5	2.5	1.8
Average	4.04	3.76	3.54	3.25	3.17

Source: U.S. Bureau of the Census, *Census of the Population, Current Population Reports: Household and Family Characteristics,* Series P-20, Number 407 (Washington, D.C.: GPO, 1992).

families are more taxed than those in the past (Hobbs et al. 1984; Moroney 1986), the new challenges that they face are imposing, to be sure.

The size of the average American family dropped by 20 percent, or by almost one person, between 1930 and 1990. Sixty years ago, one in three families had five or more members; in 1990 only one in seven families was that large. In 1990, 40 percent of *all* families were composed of only two people, compared with 26 percent in 1930.

Even though women have married earlier in each successive generation since the turn of the century and theoretically were increasingly more likely to have more children, the birth rate has actually declined between 1900 and 1990 despite a swing upward between 1950 and 1960. The average number of children seventy-five years ago was 2.9 per family; in 1990 it was 2.2. Such a trend has had a significant impact on family structure and family life. For example, in the middle of the last century, the average mother was still bearing children well into her forties; by 1900, she had completed her childbearing functions at thirty-three; and by 1980 the age had dropped to twenty-nine. Unlike her forebears, today's mother is likely to have completed her child-rearing functions in her forties (although a small but significant number of career women are postponing childbearing until their thirties and are raising their children in their forties).

The reasons for such changes are numerous. As a society becomes more industrialized, for example, it develops social security and social insurance systems. In the past, many parents viewed their children, however

TABLE 2.4. Female Labor Force Participation Rates (in Percentages), 1950–1990

Age	1950	1960	1970	1980	1990
16–19	41.0	39.4	44.0	51.8	55.2
20–24	46.1	46.2	57.8	68.4	75.2
25–34	34.0	36.0	45.0	57.4	63.5
35–44	39.1	43.5	51.1	58.3	63.0
45–54	38.0	49.8	54.4	57.1	60.3
55–64	27.0	37.2	43.0	41.9	42.3
Total	33.9	37.8	43.4	48.4	51.4

Sources: U.S. Department of Labor, *Employment and Earnings Statistics,* vol. 40, no. 1 (Washington, D.C.: GPO, 1993); C. Taeuber, ed., *Statistical Handbook on Women in America* (Phoenix: Oryx Press, 1991).

erroneously, as their old-age insurance—the greater the number of children, the greater the insurance (Schottland 1963). With the availability of collective social insurance mechanisms, the need for large families has diminished. Changes in medical and social practices have also contributed to a dramatic reduction in infant mortality rates. When these rates were extraordinarily high, the norm was to have a large number of pregnancies on the assumption that only a few children would survive. For example, estimates are that one hundred years ago, one child in five died before reaching the age of one, and one in three died before reaching his or her fifth year. Additionally, fertility control measures have increased in both availability and reliability.

Women's roles and expectations have also changed significantly over the past fifty years, furthering the trend toward smaller families. In the past, women had fewer opportunities for careers outside the home, and prior to World War II, mothers experienced heavy societal pressure not to work outside the home. Since that time, economic realities have encouraged women both to seek employment and to limit the size of their families (see table 2.4). Large families are now viewed as a barrier to social mobility and to a higher standard of living, and mothers, many of whom have completed their childbearing function by age thirty, have the time, the opportunity, and often the need to begin or resume careers outside the home.

In 1900, 20 percent of women between the ages of sixteen and sixty-four were employed. Over the next forty years, the rate gradually rose to

26 percent. The figures for married women rose from slightly less than 5 to 15 percent during the same period. Older women, ages forty-five to sixty-four, were less likely to be a part of the labor force—14 percent in 1900 and 20 percent in 1940.

The trend accelerated over the next fifty years: 50 percent of all women are now employed, and married women living with their husbands make up 57 percent of the female labor force. Whereas women's rate of participation in the labor force increased by 36 percent between 1960 and 1990, the labor force participation rate for married women has increased by 68 percent, and for mothers with children under the age of six, by 62 percent. Almost one-half of women with children under age six now work outside their homes.

However necessary and enabling these changes may be, they have created new and unanticipated pressures on today's families, one of which involves the growing need for caretaking among the elderly. Whereas children were likely to be the largest group of dependents in earlier years (for example, in 1910 there were twelve children for every elderly person), both children and grandparents today often look to the family for care (for instance, in 1990 there were only three children for every elderly person).

This shift in the dependency ratio is creating new pressures for families and especially for mothers (see table 2.5). It is not simply a matter of transferring care from children to elderly parents, because for most families there is a significant hiatus between periods of caretaking need. Mothers who have completed their childbearing during their twenties may be faced with the responsibility of tending to aged parents fifteen to twenty years after their children have become independent, necessitating major lifestyle adjustments. Further adjustments are required because of the differences in children's and elderly adults' caregiving needs. The adaptations incumbent on today's families who care for aging parents are more significant than in decades past when there were proportionately fewer elderly people, more unemployed women, and higher percentages of unmarried women residing within the households of their nuclear or extended families. These women were expected to take the role of caregiver. Those between the ages of forty-five and fifty-four were looked to in particular, as they represented the generation immediately following the elderly group.

While the reality of this fact has not been contested, a growing number of researchers have pointed out that informal care, especially "family" care, really means care provided by women. This reality has proven problematic for these researchers. One group has suggested that women are not given the recognition they deserve for the significant contributions they make not only to other family members but also to society in the sense that they provide this care without financial reimbursement. The other views this reality as unacceptable in the sense that women are being exploited by a patriarchal society. Given this, the only solution is to stop providing the care so that society in general and men in particular will be forced to change. (For examples of these arguments, see Ungerson 1987; Land and Rose 1985; and Wilson 1977.) We agree with these critiques. However, we would hope that a solution to the problem need not involve the more radical position of the latter.

In 1900, for every one hundred elderly persons in the population, there were ninety-seven women in the age grouping forty-five to fifty-four, of whom eight were single/never married—close to a 1:1 ratio. Fifty years later, this ratio had dropped sharply, and by 1990 there were only forty-six women aged forty-five to fifty-four for every one hundred persons over sixty-four. During this period (1900–1990), the elderly population increased by 185 percent and the percentage of women aged forty-five to fifty-four by only 35 percent. Shifts in the single/never married group are even more striking. Whereas there were almost eight single women for every one hundred elderly persons, there are now only two, an overall reduction of 71 percent.

This pool of potential caregivers has shrunk throughout the century. More than 60 percent of all women in the age group forty-five to fifty-four and over 40 percent of all women aged fifty-five to sixty-four are in the labor force. Moreover, 86 percent of married women between the ages of forty-five and sixty-four are working outside the home. The rates for single women in these age groups are even higher. These women, once a major source of caregiving, are either unavailable entirely for caregiving activities or are performing both employment and caregiving functions.

The declining caregiving ratios, shown in table 2.5, are striking.

Another characteristic of the modern family that affects its capacity to provide care is the growing divorce rate. It has been projected that 40–50 percent of all marriages of women born between 1940 and 1944, for example, will end in divorce and that one in two children born in the 1970s will see their parents divorce or will experience the death of a parent before they reach eighteen years of age, facts that are attributable to changes in attitudes and liberalization of divorce laws (Goode 1975). Al-

TABLE 2.5. Caregiver and Dependency Ratios, 1900–1990

Year	Elderly Population (%)	Women 45–54 (%)	Rate/1,000	Ratios, Single/Never Married Women, 45–54/1,000 Elderly
1900	4.07	3.83	966	76
1910	4.31	4.20	974	83
1920	4.63	4.55	983	94
1930	5.45	5.10	937	84
1940	6.81	5.72	837	72
1950	8.14	5.73	708	55
1960	9.23	5.78	625	44
1970	9.80	5.88	600	29
1980	10.5	5.73	561	25
1990	11.6	5.16	456	22

Sources: U.S. Bureau of the Census, *Historical Statistics of the United States: From Colonial Times to 1957* (Washington, D.C.: GPO, 1960), 23–25; U.S. Bureau of the Census, *Census of Population: Current Population Reports, Household and Family Characteristics,* Series P-20, Number 467 (Washington, D.C.: GPO, 1992).

though most Americans feel that divorce is preferable to an unhappy marriage (Yankelovich, Skelly, and White 1977), divorce still brings stress to those involved and impairs the family's ability to provide care (Hetherington, Cox, and Cox 1977; Schorr and Moen 1977). For instance, most single-parent families live in poverty, and 85 percent of all divorced women are unemployed, as compared with an employment rate of 51 percent for women in general.

Although most children do live in a home with a mother and a father, the proportion of children under six who lived with both parents declined from 87.5 percent in 1960 to 71 percent in 1990; the number of children living only with their mothers increased from five million to almost fifteen million. The trend toward an increasing number of single-parent families is likely to continue throughout the remainder of this century.

Despite the increasingly complex demands placed on family members and the continuing pattern of stress and limited support, families—in the American tradition, especially their women members—are expected to carry out the caregiving tasks for their own family members and, as individuals, to be available to provide care to nonfamily members as volunteers as if they were automatically capable and autonomous. There is mounting evidence, however, that this expectation is unrealistic. As a result, families providing care need resources and supports to permit adequate family functioning and adequate fulfillment of the special needs of their members with disabilities, because these families often experience significant stress that goes beyond what is considered to be "normal" in a family system. They are, consequently, placed at risk for systemic difficulty and burnout because too often the larger society and its formal caregiving system have not adapted to the needs of today's families. An employed single parent, for example, may have problems in interacting with external social service agencies because their hours of operation conflict with her work schedule, and families providing care to disabled members may experience difficulties associated with a social welfare system that is not attuned to their complex needs.

Although it is clear that there is not a single prototype of families caring for members with disabilities, our society has not recognized or accepted the viability of many family types. A number of types can be described, but categorizing families in a detailed manner would not be productive for establishing more effective social policy, because to do so is to assume that most families are static. A more realistic approach is to recognize and analyze the fluidity of families and their structure, functions, and changes over time. There are periods in the family life cycle, for example, in which the father tends to be the sole wage earner as the mother cares for the children at home. This stage may be relatively short-lived when the total family life course is analyzed. Transitional phases and other changes in family conditions are common and need to be understood as such.

Caregiving: A Recapitulation and an Agenda

Schorr (1968) has offered one of the more reasoned statements on the issue of the changing nature of families: "The flat statement that the family . . . is deteriorating cannot be supported. The family is changing. Some of the changes may be bad and others are all to the good" (133). This is the key. All social institutions change, the family among them. Today's society is not yesterday's. There have been significant improvements in the overall quality of life for most people (for example, in the areas of mortality, morbidity, longevity, education, and employment conditions). These improvements, however, have been accompanied by changes in the economic system whereby individuals and families face new demands that previous families were not required to meet.

There is an American tendency to establish dichotomies, to argue that *either* the formal *or* the informal caregiving system should assume primary responsibility in meeting the needs of persons with disabilities. For example, thirty years ago, professionals advised families with children with severe disabilities to place them in institutions. It was better for the child; it was better for other children in the family; it was better for the parents. Those parents who wanted to keep the child at home were told they lacked the skills, knowledge, and resources required by the child to reach his or her potential. Many ambivalent parents were made to feel guilty if they resisted the recommended institutional care.

Recently, however, the pendulum has swung to the opposite side. Professionals now typically believe that community care, including family care, is superior to institutional care. The current thinking is that institutional care is not in the best interest of the child or the family as a whole. There have been exceptions to these polar positions, but we have a tendency to see solutions in either/or terms rather than to accept the value of diversity and interdependency between the informal and the formal caregiving systems. It is clear that in some instances the formal system is in a position to provide better care; and in others the informal system is in a better position to be the primary caregiver. And, of course, we need to recognize the benefits of both being involved at the same time in some instances. Within this framework, both systems are important, and neither should be seen as preferable over the other.

The formal system, that is, public and private health, social welfare, and related agencies, cannot take over one of the most basic of human functions—the provision of emotional support, affection, and love. Some caregiving functions carried out by families, friends, neighbors, and volunteers in the broadest sense can be provided for by the formal system— for example, the giving of physical care, whether this involves the provision of meals, housekeeping, a place to live, recreation, and income maintenance. What we need to move toward is an interdependent system, a single system, combining the informal and formal systems, one that is based on a sense of shared responsibility. The essence of sharing, of course, is a recognition by the formal system that families, friends, and others make a considerable contribution and that historical ideas of professional turf and unilateral relationships need to give way to the higher level ideal of "exchange" and mutual respect among all caregivers.

With a clear understanding of family fluidity, it becomes easy to see that all families—from diverse backgrounds and living in a variety of life circumstances—are at risk and that these changes over time bring about periods of greater and lesser need for external support systems. Caregiving heightens this risk. What are the issues? What has been society's response?

In the next several chapters, we examine key issues related to the ability of the existing human services system to engage in caregiving that aspires to be caring. In this examination, we identify major obstacles that we must address if this system is to become responsive.

3 ～   The Professional Response

ED ROSENBAUM's book *A Taste of My Own Medicine* (1988) became an extraordinary film in the hands of director Randa Haines. *The Doctor,* released in 1991, portrays a heart surgeon, Doctor Jack MacKee. Handsome, witty, and of undeniable skill—the envy of the residents, the hospital staff, and his physician partners—Jack is the epitome of the technically rational expert: the doctor knows best; the patient should comply; competent surgical cutting is obviously better than caring healing. Jack's initial understanding of his professional duty is that the choice facing the physician between competence and caring is an either/or matter and that technical rationality makes competence the obvious preference. In almost classically tragic fashion, the gods reward Jack's arrogance by dealing him a potentially mortal blow.

He develops cancer of the throat, which doesn't respond to initial treatment and requires surgery. While dealing with this life-threatening illness, Jack angrily experiences the bureaucratized and alienating structures of the medical system: being asked to fill out endless redundant forms; being treated as a case, not a person; being mechanically processed through test after test, specialist after specialist. He finally dismisses from his case a technically rational physician, a woman whose manner reminds us of Jack himself, and chooses instead a caring surgeon, a man who had formerly been the object of Jack's derision because of his "soft" and caring approach to medicine. Through his own experiences as a patient, Jack comes to realize that he himself has been a primary contributor to the uncaring medical world and, worse yet, has been helping to socialize young physicians into a way of practice virtually lacking caring. He learns that caring and competence are not antithetical. In fact, he comes to believe that one cannot be an effective healer without caring.

In that regard, consider this quote from a leading physician reported by Schreiber (1993): "I think 99.9 percent of people who enter medicine do so because they want to help people, and it's almost as if we beat it out of a lot of them over time. When I went to med school . . . in the sixties, it was a reign of terror; we were terrified and we hurt a lot and we probably took that out on our patients. But I think what's coming into medicine now is a loud, focused cry from patients saying, 'you guys better care more. We're people'" (148). Apparently many medical schools are hearing this message and increasingly incorporating caring into the curriculum.

Several other recent American films have portrayed the problems of those who care for others. *Rain Man,* for example, depicts a brash young man blindly pursuing material things to the point of crass insensitivity to the needs of his long-lost brother who has autism. He learns a series of hard lessons about himself and the humanity and value of people through eventually coming to care for this strange but endearing person. They both make major strides as human beings as they overcome the challenges posed by a world in which caring is not a priority. The film affords a dramatic example of Mayeroff's (1971) claim for the mutual benefit to caregiver and care recipient in a truly caring relationship.

In another recent film, *Regarding Henry,* we see a high-powered, fast-lane lawyer who deals impersonally and uncaringly with all the people in his life—clients, colleagues, family members, even himself. Only after he is seriously wounded as an innocent bystander in a robbery does he begin to question his value system and his way of relating to people. A caring therapist, who helps him recover from his debilitating injuries, and his concerned family members help him begin to alter his perspective. We come to see through his eyes that careerism, with its excessive emphasis on competition and the use of power to manipulate people, turns one into an uncaring, unethical, unfeeling exploiter—ironically, a victim of the system. But note, this insight is very difficult to come by. As with Jack MacKee in *The Doctor,* it took a life-threatening condition to enlighten Henry. Short of such an experience, the film suggests, we are so caught up in the dehumanization of contemporary society that we remain blind to what it does to us.

Why is caring so difficult in our society? The many recent films challenging our tendency to treat others as things to be manipulated for our own purposes, rather than as persons deserving our care, suggest that Hollywood views this as an important question on the minds of the public. Although not widely discussed, the challenge of caring, we argue in this book, is central to our life together in society.

Barriers within the Formal Caring System

The professions are in crisis.[1] Professional persons—perhaps especially those who want to be caring—are harried and perpetually short of time, beleaguered, beset by regulations and cost-cutting proposals, and out of favor in the media and among many segments of the public. Said Schön (1983): "Professionals claim to contribute to social well-being, put their clients' needs ahead of their own, and hold themselves accountable to standards of competence and morality. But both popular and scholarly critics accuse the professions of serving themselves at the expense of their clients, ignoring their obligations to public service, and failing to police themselves effectively" (11–12).

Criticisms such as Schön's have, if anything, grown in number and stridency over the last ten years. The crisis of the professions is one of legitimacy and of self- and public confidence, shared by the professions with most of society's major institutions—government, the military, religion, education, and corporate business. The professional crisis has its own dynamics, however, with prominent ethical features. Many professionals have lost touch with the major reason for their practice, their ethical center, namely, to foster the human development of their clients through caring and thereby to enhance community and the common good.

Toward Reflective Practice

To further our understanding of the nature of caring and the many obstacles it faces in contemporary society, it is helpful to investigate the nature of professional roles. Caring for clients in today's world requires a fundamental professional role reassessment. This is what Donald Schön (1983) has called for in *The Reflective Practitioner*. Schön describes two very different models of professional roles: technical rationality (Model I) and reflective practice (Model II).[2]

Technical rationality, for Schön, is "the model that is embedded in the institutional context of professional life" (25). The major professional role in technical rationality is problem solving. Technically rational professionals give little attention to the value-laden task of problem setting—the "process by which we define decisions, ends and means" (39) within particular contexts. A danger clearly inherent in this technically rational approach to caregiving is arbitrarily molding the practice situation to conform to professional knowledge. Professional practice often becomes a Procrustean bed in which the client is trimmed or stretched to fit the professional's understanding.

The professional assumes the role of the expert, the one who knows all. The expectation is that clients will "put themselves in the professionals' hands and comply completely with their advice" (302). Technical rationality describes the traditional treatment-focused, top-down approach to caregiving in professional practice: professionals have all the power and all the answers; their role is to "fix" or cure the individual client. As one professional caregiver commented: "Family members should carry out doctors orders. The family doesn't understand or doesn't know enough to understand. Some families try to do too much without the doctors orders. Have more meetings together with handouts to help give instructions."

In contrast, *reflective practice* entails reframing both the professional's and the client's role expectations. Reflective practice calls for complementarity: the client and the professional enter a partnership in which caregiving entails caring and joint exploration of the situation. The professional has expertise yet realizes that this knowledge is incomplete without the unique perspective of the client. The professional's relationship with the client "takes on the form of a reflective conversation, where the reflective practitioner tries to discover the limits of his expertise" (300) instead of imposing predetermined knowledge upon the client. Another professional caregiver, recognizing the two-sided nature of the caregiving transaction, said, "The family should get as much information as possible, read, research and ask questions. The professional should get as much education as possible, read, research, continue to get education. We have much to learn from listening to one another."

The reflective practitioner enters transactions with clients possessing some expert knowledge and a theory of professional practice. Unlike the technically rational professional, however, the reflective practitioner does not assume the traditional expert role. Instead, caregiving entails a reflective and caring relationship with the client that involves exploring multiple perspectives and sharing responsibility for both problem setting and problem solving. This client-professional partnership "incorporates recognition of the autonomy of those being served but also includes solidarity with them" (Lebacqz 1985, 57). In that spirit, a caregiver suggested simply, "The professional should be a nice person. Don't be so professional. Be friendly and respect the other person and provide information."

TABLE 3.1. Contrasting Professional Perspectives

Technically Rational Expert (Model I)	Reflective Practitioner (Model II)
I am presumed to know and must claim to do so, regardless of my own uncertainty.	I am presumed to know, but I am not the only one in the situation to have relevant knowledge. My uncertainties may be a source of learning for me and for them.
Keep my distance from the client and hold onto the expert's role. Give the client a sense of my expertise but convey a feeling of warmth and sympathy as a "sweetener."	Seek out connections to the client's thoughts and feelings. Allow his respect for my knowledge to emerge from this discovery of it in the situation.
Look for deference and status in the client's response to my professional persona.	Look for the sense of freedom and of real connection to the client, as a consequence of no longer needing to maintain a professional facade.

Source: Schön 1983, 300.

For caregiving to become caring, many professionals must move from the more typical technical rationality to reflective practice. This will require changes of perspective, not only on their part but by clients as well. The following two tables, adapted from Schön, depict the changes in outlook required for the professional's move from technically rational expert caregiver to caring reflective practitioner and for the client's move from the traditional technically rational contract to the reflective contract.

The contrasting professional perspectives on the client-professional transaction depicted in table 3.1 suggest the need for significant, personally demanding change. Technical rationality's all-knowing, objectively distant, and status-conscious caregiving role would be shifted to reflective practice's appreciation for the limits of one's knowledge, a caring relation with the client as a person at both intellectual and feeling levels, and more genuine, less status-directed relationships.

Many clients may be intimidated and/or frustrated by reflective practitioners. As suggested in table 3.2, they have been socialized into a role of having faith in professionals and wanting them to guarantee security, being unquestioningly compliant, and expecting unerring professional expertise and caregiving.

TABLE 3.2. Contrasting Client Perspectives

Traditional Rational Contract (Model I)	Reflective Contract (Model II)
I put myself into the professional's hands, and in doing this, I gain a sense of security based on faith.	I join with the professional in making sense of my case, and in doing this I gain a sense of increased involvement and action.
I have the comfort of being in good hands. I need only comply with his advice and all will be well.	I can exercise some control over the situation. I am not wholly dependent on him; he is also dependent on information and action that only I can undertake.
I am pleased to be served by the best person available.	I am pleased to be able to test my judgments about his competence. I enjoy the excitement of discovery about his knowledge, about the phenomena of his practice, and about myself.

Source: Schön 1983, 302.

A relationship with a professional built on client participation, interdependence, and discovery will require some getting used to, and this in turn will require the professional to be willing to engage in mutual learning and exploration with the client in the process of caregiving. It should be obvious that changed modes of professional and public education will also be necessary to produce this more caring professional way of caregiving.

Toward Partnership and Shared Responsibility

Two terms come to mind in considering challenges to client and professional role expectations in pursuit of caring, namely, *partnership* and *shared responsibility*. Dunst, Trivette, and Deal (1988) address the first in arguing that "partnerships are valued over paternalistic approaches because the former implies and conveys the belief that partners are capable individuals who become more capable by sharing knowledge, skills, and resources in a manner that leaves all participants better off after entering into a cooperative arrangement" (9). Observed one caregiver, "More effort should be made to pull the family into the process (if the client agrees). We try to be all things to all people and we're not here for that. Many things can be provided if we connect with the right family member. We get into the role of, 'I'm the professional caregiver and I know what the client needs.' You can pick up little things that make a difference from family and other supporters."

This emphasis on partnership is complemented by Moroney (1986) in *Shared Responsibility*. Moroney makes the idea of need central to his analysis of family social policy. He illustrated his notion of shared responsibility with an account of an incident, worth quoting here at length. While on a visit to the United Kingdom, Moroney

> accompanied a local authority social worker carrying out a survey of handi-
> capped persons. An elderly couple, the husband 80 years old and disabled
> from a stroke, the wife caring for him despite severe arthritis, was asked in the
> course of the interview what needs they had and what problems the local so-
> cial services agency might help them with. By any number of standards, the
> couple had many professionally defined needs. They lived in a second story
> flat with the toilet in the backyard. The apartment was heated by a single fire-
> place and three space heaters. They were able to move about with difficulty
> but were visited by their neighbors. The couple told the social worker that they
> would like some assistance. The wife pointed to a large tree outside the bed-
> room window and said that they were worried that a large overhanging branch
> might strike the window and break it. If this were to happen in the winter,
> they might freeze to death. Neither she, her husband, nor the neighbors could
> do anything about it, and she wondered if the social worker could arrange to
> have the branch cut off. The professional response was not atypical: "That's
> fine, but let's talk about your real needs." (155–156)

In this illustration, the clients had a keen understanding of their needs. The professional, however, was enacting a caregiving role that made him insensitive to his clients and virtually incapable of caring. Although not at issue in this incident, professional insensitivity can be particularly prob-lematic where the use and abuse of professional power are concerned.

Professional Power

Society vests professionals with power.[3] Professional power is "legitimated and institutionalized power" (Lebacqz 1985, 113). Professionals do not simply have the power to fix a problem. They also define its reality. Distortion and abuse are possible depending upon the way professionals use their reality-defining power. They may use it in the service of caring or for their own, decidedly uncaring purposes.

Craig and Craig (1973) describe two very different views of power, labeled *directive* and *synergic*[4]—based on whether we respect others as persons or see them merely as objects. Directive power often characterizes technically rational experts' preferred mode of caregiving. They often use their expert power to exercise control over the client. In doing so, they make the client dependent and powerless: "Directive power dehumanizes people because it makes them less sensitive to the fact that they cause the results of their actions" (61). It reduces their belief in their own self-efficacy. Directive power, however, is the sort of power embedded within the structures of society and professional practice and caregiving. If we approach clients exercising this typical form of power, we will rarely care for, enable, or empower them.

In contrast to directive power, synergic power suggests a very different use of professional power. Synergic power is "the capacity of an individual to increase the satisfaction of all participants by intentionally generating increased energy and creativity, all of which is used to *co-create* a more rewarding present and future" (62). In accordance with this model, clients are colleagues and allies with whom professionals join in a cooperative and caring relationship, as in reflective practice. Synergic power grows from openness and trust. Its ultimate goals are (a) to enhance people's senses of autonomy and interdependence that grow out of working together, (b) to enhance people's view of themselves as able to affect their own and others' destiny, (c) to enhance people's view of others as able to work together, and (d) to facilitate caring and thereby human development. Synergic power is an alternative to the traditional view of the professional caregiver as controlling expert, and it is this type of power that caring professionals would employ to enhance clients' human development and self-efficacy.

This idea of synergic power also relates to issues raised by Lebacqz (1985, 131) about the societal distribution of power with the goal of client empowerment or liberation. Caring requires that professionals redistribute power through sharing it, yet we encounter a complex paradox in notions such as empowerment and liberation. If professionals assume that their role is to empower or liberate clients, they may veer uncomfortably close to paternalism. Empowerment and liberation sometimes become directive when they imply that clients passively experience professional benevolence. The professional's use of power in caregiving, therefore, must involve synergic efforts—professional and client working cooperatively to achieve results greater than either one could achieve alone.

The reflective practitioner does not ask, "What can *I do* for this client?" but "How would the client's empowerment happen here?" Caring requires synergic rather than directive transactions, since they have a much greater chance of addressing clients' real needs and priorities, equalizing the distribution of power, and promoting human development.

Communication

A key task of a caring client-professional transaction that embodies reflective practice and synergic power type is understanding and defining the client's personal *projects*.[5] Personal projects are the overarching schemes or plans that give shape to our lives. They are the narratives we enact, complete with goals, intentions, and motivations. They are what get us up in the morning and give direction to our striving. The key to understanding projects lies in client-professional communication within the caregiving situation. Simply, said one caregiver, we "should talk with family to find out likes and dislikes. There is not enough communication. We need to work together more." Said another, "Professionals need to listen to parents more often and trust their information."

Critical theory, as proposed by Habermas and the Frankfurt school (Habermas 1971, 1973, 1975), provides a means for analyzing communication in pursuit of caring. Critical theory seeks the ideal of "uncoerced consensus and non-manipulated understanding and agreement" (Forrester 1983, 238). The idea is that we should judge situations based on the degree to which they manifest valid, truly free, and authentic communication. This ideal relates to synergic power and reflective practice in emphasizing that we should work together to formulate professional action, not impose interventions upon clients. It also provides a means for both the caregivers and clients to come to know their situation, which is central to the caring transaction. Critical theory identifies obstacles that impede communication and prevent clients and caregivers—and all caring and cared-for persons—from jointly exploring client projects and meanings and the caring actions related to them.

According to the model of communication in critical theory (Habermas 1973), we must consider claims to the validity of what speakers say and listeners hear. Listeners evaluate four claims in what they hear speakers say: (1) truth—the existence or factual quality of an aspect of the world being spoken about; (2) legitimacy—the appropriateness of what they hear in the context in which they hear it; (3) sincerity—whether they believe the speaker means and intends to say what she is saying; and (4) clarity—how understandable and coherent is what is being said.

Acceptance of these communicative claims has pragmatic results. The claim to truth engenders belief, legitimacy engenders consent, sincerity engenders trust, and clarity engenders attention. Simply put, we should strive to create situations in which the parties can believe, consent to, trust, attend to, and thereby comprehend what each other communicates. When these claims are distorted, misinformation and manipulation may result. Several examples of these communicative claims and their violation can be drawn from the domain of early-intervention caregiving with families of children with developmental disabilities (Sokoly and Dokecki 1992).

> When early intervention caregivers do not give parents honest information about their child's condition and deny developmental concerns that do exist, argue Sokoly and Dokecki, the *claim to truth* is invalidated. When parents see delays in development that call into question their beliefs about their child's normality, they begin to doubt any information they receive from the caregiver. This has negative effects on the parent-caregiver relationship since channels of communication and discourse have broken down. *Caring requires that communication be true.*
>
> The *claim of legitimacy* involves issues such as whether caregivers have sufficient valid information about child and family resources, priorities, concerns, and projects that is adequate for planning effective early interventions. While parents might agree to illegitimate recommendations, they are often unable to carry them out. The result is frustration and a lack of developmental change. *Caring requires that communication be legitimate.*
>
> If we do not uphold the claim of sincerity, we cannot maintain cooperation and trust. Attempts by caregivers to manipulate information and misguide parents' judgments about their children invalidate this claim. *Caring requires that communication be sincere.*

Finally, the *claim to clarity* relates to whether caregivers communicate with parents in readily understandable, jargon-free language. If this is not so, parents leave the caregiver's office feeling confused and frustrated.

Caring Requires That Communication Be Clear

In contrast to these examples, honoring claims to communication can lead to a caring and authentic partnership and produce more effective caregiving interventions. Because of the importance of upholding the validity of communicative claims, free and uncoerced communication should characterize transactions of clients and caring professionals. "As discourse is denied to participants, they are likely to be rendered dependent, powerless, ignorant, and mystified" (Forrester 1983, 240). This suggests that true empowerment involves eliminating socially unnecessary distortions in communication between clients and caregivers. Forrester asserts that some distortions—those that are accidental, unforeseeable, and just plain human—are bound to occur. Other distortions, however, are neither natural nor humanly and socially necessary and, as a result, are avoidable. Avoidable and preventable distortions most likely occur when caregivers assume an imperious expert role, are insensitive and impersonal, ignore differences based on gender, ethnic group membership, and the like, and use directive power to exert control over clients, in other words, act in a decidedly uncaring fashion.

In pursuit of avoiding and preventing communicative distortions so as to enhance the likelihood that caregiving is truly caring, we now turn to an examination of the nature of service delivery and discuss how the nature of the relationships between formal and informal caregivers as well as the dynamics of the relationships between caregivers and care recipients can facilitate or impede their accessing needed supportive services.

4~ Barriers to Caregiving Services and Caring Relationships

T HUS FAR, we have presented fundamental issues central to caring and caregiving. In chapter 1, we developed the argument that caring—actions that promote the mutual human development of caregiver and care recipient—is the ideal form of caregiving. In chapter 2, we discussed the needs and characteristics of those needing services, the contributions that families and other informal caregivers are making, and the demands they experience by virtue of giving care. In chapter 3, we examined the nature of the relationship between formal and informal caregivers and concluded that significant communication problems often exist in their relationships.

The many issues identified so far, however, are only a part of the overall challenge we must face if we are to move toward becoming a more caring society with effective caregivers who are truly caring. The purpose of this chapter is to identify and discuss additional facets of the caregiving situation.

Stress and Caregiving

Caregiving is a human service transaction that is built on a relationship between caregivers and care recipients. There is a process of communication through which resources are transferred and through which the emotional process of caring develops.

Spending time in close quarters with good communication is expected to yield interpersonal bonds that will lead to caring commitments and markedly improved caregiving services. One hopefully starts from a good foundation with family members, for there is already a social/psychological bond, but it is often undermined by the poor communication and unresolved feelings. To the extent that good communication can be achieved and maintained, this problem could be markedly decreased.

These stressors occur as a result of the various personal characteristics coming together in each of the caregiving transactions. They primarily relate to communication skills, but there are contextual aspects to consider as well. The purpose of this categorization is to emphasize the fact that there are many interactions and interrelationships that must be focused on when considering the transactional nature of the caregiving situation. In Mullan's (1993) stress framework, he refers to the caregiving context as including such aspects of the relationship as the history, quality, and amount of time as caregiver. Matthews (1993) includes aspects such as the frequency, timing, and duration of the caregiving transaction that serve as barriers to caregiving. This categorization of barriers is to make the point that the quality of the interactions resulting from a caregiving relationship can have direct impact on the success of the transactions.

Biegel et al. (1991) proposed that the nature of the prognosis and the patient's characteristics play large roles in determining the success of the caregiving transactions. For example, one woman interviewed for the CARE-NET study recalled that she had always loved and admired her husband for being so kind, loving, and committed to his family. With the onset of his illness, though, these characteristics were replaced with demanding, critical, and cross attitudes. She was scared to criticize him because his chances of recovery were very low, and she did not want to help him realize how much he was changing. This example emphasizes the need for the emotional services discussed earlier, such as support groups, and also the need for instrumental services, such as general information about how illnesses can affect one's mental, as well as physical, health.

It is important to note that some of these relational issues can affect the degree to which the caregiver will experience burnout with the caregiving situation. Specific aspects such as frequency, timing, and duration of the caregiving role and the prognosis of the care recipient can influence how the caregiver perceives the situation. Burnout, in turn, can be a barrier in itself, in that it has a negative impact on the utilization of formal services (Stephens 1993). The potential for burnout is rather clear in the following account of one woman's history as an informal caregiver:

I have been caring for my elderly mother for about 12 years now. During these years, my brother and sister also lived with me, at different times, because they needed my care to help them fight cancer; they have since died of cancer. Before they lived in my home, my step-father was with me for the first 18 months my mother was here, until he died of heart disease. I don't know how much longer my mother will be with me; I suppose until she is also gone.

Stress and strain are affected by physical health, age, ethnicity, coping strategies, and perceived stress (manifested as depression, anger, and/or frustration). The notion that competing role demands act as barriers to the provision of services has been widely acknowledged (Avison et al. 1993; Biegel et al. 1991; Edwards 1990; Gilbert 1973; Goldfarb et al. 1986). Competing role demands (Biegel et al. 1991; Mullan 1993; Matthews 1993) can come in the form of other caregiving roles in the family, such as the number of children in the household, or the amount of time the caregivers must spend working in situations not concerning the care recipient. Other major life events occurring at the same time one is involved in the caregiving relationships increase the competing role demands. In determining the impact of family contexts and experiences on caregiving, Avison et al. (1993) found that life events have a large contributing effect on the amount of distress among caregivers and, hence, their utilization of services.

Psychological strains (Mullan 1993) are manifested in feelings of overload, anxiety, anger, or depression. It is important to understand that these strains, which often serve as barriers to the utilization of services (Stephens 1993), tend to be the culmination of some of the other personal factors, such as competing role demands, physical health, age, and ethnicity, but can also be caused by more subjective factors such as one's perception of stress or availability of coping strategies. Stephens (1993) stresses the role that subjective factors can play in one's ability to function within caregiving relationships. In asserting that personal characteristics such as health, age, and ethnicity can serve as barriers to caregiving, we are emphasizing the role that these factors play in contributing to intrapsychic strains, perception of stress, and use of coping strategies.

The following story illustrates how such intrapsychic strains, lack of a sense of mastery, poor physical health, and age can interrelate to form a barrier for this informal caregiver's attempt to care for his wife:

Because of the stress caused by caring for my wife who has a mental disorder, and the fact that I am not a young man and do not have time to care for myself, I have developed a number of health problems. I know that these are not only physical health problems, but are also related to the guilt that I feel because of this situation, which I know I did not cause; but, still, I also know that I have no control and cannot bring her back to me. I am no longer able to care for her as I used to.

Needs of Caregivers and Care Recipients

As we have already seen, caregivers experience varying degrees of stress that can become overpowering if ignored. We must therefore explore what is it about caregiving that is problematic, difficult to handle, and thus stressful. In that regard, we will identify the specific, concrete needs of caregivers and consider interventions to address these needs.

The development of caregiving has a natural history. Care recipients come to the place where they cannot care for themselves independently and turn to others to help meet their basic needs. This is an informal process usually undertaken by family members or significant others in their lives. Informal caregivers often decide that they need some external resources to do their job properly. They seek contact with the formal service system to try to obtain those resources. This section identifies and discusses that mix of services necessary for a comprehensive service delivery system.

For the purpose of analysis, we have identified three caregiving roles: care recipient (CR), informal caregiver (IC), and formal caregiver (FC). Table 4.1 depicts traditional resources organized to reflect the caregiving transactions through which caregiving services typically occur. The table is illustrative of typical arrangements, not exhaustive regarding either the services[1] or the transactions. Obviously, the unique characteristics of each caregiving transaction will determine which specific services would apply.[2] The use of this categorization enables us to see similarities and differences between various forms of caregiving relationships and services.

Roles and Functions of Caregivers

Table 4.1 depicts six caregiving transactions, each involving two people, the one providing (left) and the one receiving (right) the caregiving services, with the arrows denoting the directionality of the provision of services.

TABLE 4.1. Services in Caregiving Relationships

	FC→CR	FC→IC	FC→FC	IC→CR	IC→IC	CR→CR
Instrumental Resources Provided						
Information (re illness, cost of services)	X	X	X	X	X	X
Assistance with activities of daily living (bathing, toileting, feeding)	X			X		
Transportation	X			X		
Home chores (cleaning, shopping)	X			X		
Day care	X					
Skilled medical (inpatient, outpatient, in-home)	X					
Respite (in-home, day care, institutional)		X	X		X	X
Financial (supplements, gifts, loans)	X	X		X		
Adaptive equipment (chairs, ramps)	X					
Adjunctive Health (speech & hearing, occupational therapy, physical therapy)	X					
Emotional/Cognitive Resources Provided						
Support groups	X	X	X	X	X	X
Counseling	X	X	X			
Psychotherapy	X	X	X			

Note: "FC" = formal caregiver; "CR" = care recipient; "IC" = informal caregiver.

The first three columns depict formal caregiving relationships. Within these relationships, formal caregivers transact with the care recipient as patient or client, primarily; with the group of family members or friends providing care for the care recipient; and with other formal caregivers. The second three columns represent informal caregiving relationships. The first of these columns depicts the caregiving relationship between an informal caregiver and a care recipient, often a family member providing care for another family member. The final two columns present two distinct but somewhat comparable transactions among like groups, those entailing informal caregivers providing supports to other informal caregivers and care recipients providing mutual support to one another. Such transactions may reflect peer-support and family-support groups, as well as the sharing of information about medical procedures, technology, services, providers, laws, and the like. Some of the activities in these transactions are formalized, such as support groups, but many are informal and often overlooked.

The delineation of caregiving services by specific relationships helps put each caregiver's role into perspective and allows each one involved in such relationships to understand the many different resources she or he provides or is expected to provide. Many of these services may not even be recognized as part of the process. For example, the first column in table 4.1—the formal caregiver providing resources to the care recipient—contains the most obvious and complete set of services, but since formal caregivers cannot provide effective and meaningful services to care recipients while ignoring the needs of the informal caregivers and the care they provide, informal roles are essential. All persons involved in the caregiving situation must realize that they have responsibilities to themselves and all others involved (whether they are formal or informal caregivers, or care recipients).

Although formal caregivers have important multiple responsibilities, the provision of caregiving services by informal caregivers is central to the caregiving process. Furthermore, as we saw in chapter 2, the importance of informal caregivers will increase in the near future as more and more people rely on family members to care for them in times of need. It is our position that it is the role of the formal caregiver to support and enhance the central caregiving function of the informal caregiver. Thus, recognition of these relationships should serve to increase caregivers' awareness of the many other transactions, besides those in which they are directly involved, that are necessary for the entire caregiving network to be a success (Gray 1990).

Services: Providing Resources and Supports

Formal and informal caregivers provide some of the same resources. The major difference between these groups concerns the degree to which certain formal services require highly technical skills or official sanction, such as a license. Although the number of services provided by informal as compared with formal caregivers is fewer in table 4.1, this does not mean that informal caregivers provide less care than formal caregivers. Indeed, informal caregivers actually provide more services than professionals even though professionals provide a broader range of services. The study of long-term care for the elderly conducted by the United States General Accounting Office (1988, 242) found that of the more than six million elderly people who depended on others for help, four out of five lived in the community and received most of their care from unpaid sources, such as family members. Only about 5 percent relied totally on paid services. Our point is not that one form of caregiving is more or less important than the other. Rather, each is important in its own way.

The provision of resources through services depicted in table 4.1 falls into two general types: instrumental and emotional/cognitive. *Instrumental* services provide resources needed to do something, to attain a goal or solve a problem. The instrumental category encompasses traditional types of caregiving services, such as physical help (walking, getting in and out of bed or up and down stairs); help with paperwork and financial matters; other practical help (preparing meals, doing shopping, housework); keeping the care recipient company; and giving medicine, injections, changing dressings (Parker 1992). This notion of instrumental is similar to what Lazarus and Folkman (1984) termed "problem-focused," in that these are services that help modify conditions so that we lessen the problems and stresses in the course of caregiving. In other words, these resources help meet concrete needs. For example, a formal caregiver may offer skilled medical services to alleviate painful symptoms caused by a disability or disease; or an informal caregiver may provide assistance in feeding and dressing.

The second type of service provides *emotional/cognitive* resources, those that are primarily supportive to the caregiving relationship. The purpose of these services is to help the caregiver and/or the care recipient cope with the situation (Lazarus and Folkman 1984). Emotional/cognitive resources help define perceptions of caregiving transactions. Through services such as social support groups, counseling, and psychotherapy, we can help support coping efforts by enabling people to understand their thoughts and feelings about the caregiving situation (Stephens 1993). These services go beyond this. They can be beneficial in preventing or resolving potential problems. For example, if a caregiver is depressed, she or he is unlikely to use the concrete services designed to alleviate many day-to-day burdensome tasks in the daily grind of providing care. This, in turn, is likely to result in depression, guilt, anger, burnout, or the like. Emotional/cognitive resources are essential to caregivers to help them cope with such psychological stresses and their related problems and make use of the instrumental services (Rein 1970).

Table 4.1 identifies ten categories of instrumental and three of emotional/cognitive resources. They are presented here to provide an orientation to what people should be able to call upon in caregiving relationships in the context of the service system.

Instrumental Resources

Services that provide instrumental resources help people meet their concrete needs. As identified in table 4.1, these resources are in the areas of information, assistance with activities of daily living, transportation, home chores, day care, skilled medical services, respite, financial assistance, adaptive equipment, and adjunctive health.

Information

American Association of Retired Persons (AARP) and Travelers Companies Foundation (1988) found that 42 percent of informal caregivers desired more information than they had on developments in medicine and health care. Informal caregivers' request for more information from formal caregivers relates directly to care recipients' need to have information about their situation, including information on the nature of the condition presented by the care recipient, what it involves, and what they might expect (that is, the prognosis). Caregivers need information on *how* to provide care (for example, techniques that can be used to assist a bedridden parent to the bathroom without physically harming themselves). Caregivers also need to have a working knowledge of community resources specific to their needs (for instance, while there might be common needs for all caregivers, those providing care for a parent with Alzheimer's disease will need different services than will parents providing care to a severely mentally handicapped child). Becoming knowledgeable about these resources involves much more than just knowing which agencies offer what services; it would also involve knowing costs and eligibility criteria.

Formal caregivers also have informational needs in many of the same areas. Although many of the informal caregivers obtain useful and realistic information from other informal caregivers and care recipients in the form of casual information exchange in caregiving settings and peer- and family-support groups, most still expect the professionals to be the primary source of information on diagnosis, prognosis, resources, and what it means in each specific instance for a particular caregiver to provide care to this particular care recipient. This latter issue will be dealt with in more detail under the section on emotional and cognitive resources.

Assistance with Activities of Daily Living

In chapter 2, we estimated that more than 6.5 million children and adults experience some degree of disability—disability that either partially or totally impedes their ability to care for themselves. Because of their disabilities, many care recipients have difficulty performing such routine tasks as walking, feeding, toileting, bathing, and dressing. Many studies (identified in chapter 2) have documented the amount of assistance provided by informal caregivers in this area and the overwhelming physical and emotional demands on informal caregivers when they provide such care. The AARP study (1988), for example, found that 68 percent of informal caregivers in their study provided assistance with at least one such activity. Kane and Penrod (1993) found that 38 percent of the care recipients they studied had three daily life activity deficiencies, and that more than 50 percent of the informal caregivers cared for them at least five hours a day.

The availability of formal caregivers such as public health nurses, visiting nurses, physical therapists, and various ancillary personnel has become extremely important as supports to both the informal caregivers and care recipients. It is not so much that these professionals take over these tasks; rather, they work with the informal caregivers so that they might become better equipped when they assist the care recipient. Coyne (1991), for example, found that the majority of calls to a community information and referral service were for assistance in this area.

Transportation

Transportation is a basic but often taken-for-granted and overlooked need. Care recipients require transportation to go not only to and from medical care services but also to stores, schools, church, day-care facilities, therapy sessions, and support group meetings. Moreover, when transportation is unavailable, these other services tend not to be used, and both the care recipient and the informal caregiver suffer, with potentially harmful results to both. While care recipients often rely on family members, neighbors, and friends for transportation (Gray 1990; Pilisuk and Parks 1988), sometimes they must seek out paid caregivers for help with this service (Lawton et al. 1989).

Home Chores

Because disabling conditions frequently keep care recipients from doing regular housecleaning, preparing meals, shopping, and the like, they typically rely on informal caregivers for help with these home chores. As with the provision of transportation, this informal caregiver service may go unnoticed because we take it for granted. The AARP (1988) survey found that formal paid caregivers also provide these services, in that informal caregivers frequently seek agencies that come to the home and do such chores.

Day-Care Services

Day-care services can help meet needs of both care recipients who require immediate supervision and informal caregivers in providing respite from demanding caregiving duties. Some service systems include day hospitalization and day service centers that serve unique groups of people with conditions such as Alzheimer's disease or mental retardation. These day-care facilities often provide other services and supports as well. For instance, care recipients may use day care to gather information about their disease or disability, and some may receive assistance with activities of daily living. In addition to these instrumental services, day care may be the means by which the care recipient receives emotional/cognitive resources, through services such as support groups, counseling, group therapy, or individual psychotherapy.

In a more general sense, day-care facilities provide opportunities for socialization that care recipients often do not receive in a residential institution or in their homes, especially since many of them live alone. Many elderly persons may no longer have a social circle because of their or their friends' debilitating conditions, which often prevent them from performing routine tasks.

Skilled Medical Services

Various types of formal caregivers provide skilled medical services in hospitals and family medical centers and in specialized facilities (for example, women's centers, ambulatory service centers, emergency rooms, skilled nursing facilities, and home health agencies). Furthermore, given the projections of greater numbers of persons with disabilities in the next century, coupled with inevitable technological advances, the need for specialized medical skills will grow. In the Nottingham et al. (1993) needs assessment, one of the highest-ranked needs expressed by formal caregivers was specialized training for existing medical personnel and an increase in the numbers of professionals with specialized training in this area.

Respite

Respite care generally involves a formal caregiver providing relief to an informal caregiver. Respite care in such a transaction takes several different forms, such as in-home care, day care, or even institutional care. What is important in respite care is not the specific type of service but the provision of resources to allow temporary relief from caregiving tasks (Caserta et al. 1987; Lawton et al. 1989). Allowing time away from routine duties can safeguard caregivers from being overloaded with the caregiving role and help prevent burnout and prevent unnecessary long-term institutionalization. In addition to formal caregivers providing respite, informal caregivers sometimes do so for one another by actions such as sitting with care recipients while caregivers take some time for themselves.

Professionals also experience burnout and potentially benefit from respite services provided by other professionals. In a recent survey of formal caregivers, Nottingham et al. (1993) found that 93 percent of the respondents claimed respite services were important to them in their work, and about half believed they needed more of these services in their communities. In that regard, Hay and Oken (1977) described an innovative program for intensive care nurses that provided a replacement nurse to be on duty to serve as a "floater." Rather than substitute for a nurse who was not present, the floater nurse would assume routine nursing responsibilities, thus allowing temporary periods of relief for other nurses. Numerous social work agencies have recognized this as a major concern and have implemented various initiatives that serve as "sabbaticals" for front-line workers in high stress positions, such as those in child protective services and hospices. These initiatives might involve being assigned temporarily to a research project, training, or another less stressful function within the agency.

Financial Resources

When family members become involved in caregiving, they more often than not find that they incur considerable expenses directly related to the provision of care (Baldwin 1985). Informal caregivers often provide money to help with the care recipient's bills. Indeed, the AARP (1988) found that 65 percent of the informal caregivers they surveyed helped care recipients with managing finances and subsidizing expenses.

In addition, Mullan (1993) introduced the important consideration of lost income—an often overlooked financial issue—in identifying the economic strain that can result from informal caregivers' lost time at work because of their caregiving activities. Indeed Biegel et al. (1991) cited the AARP (1988) finding that 33 percent of family caregivers lost time from work owing to caregiving activities.

Financial support takes many forms. The formal caregiving system provides direct financial services and supports to care recipients in the form of various income maintenance programs such as Social Security, which includes the *institutional* entitlement program (OASDI—Old Age Survivors Disability Insurance) and the *residual* means tested program (SSI—Supplemental Security Income). Although the financial support typically goes to the care recipient and not the caregiver, it is fair to assume that this money relieves some of the financial burden on the family. Other programs, although technically not income maintenance programs, also reduce some of the financial burden on the caregivers. These would include programs such as Medicare and Medicaid, which pay for some inpatient care, professional services, and community-based services such as home health care.

Adaptive Equipment

Many persons with serious health problems and disabling conditions require specialized medical and prosthetic devices (for example, life-sustaining machines, adjustable beds, wheelchairs, artificial limbs, ramps, computer-assisted aids to learning or communication) to survive and to adapt to their environment. Formal organizations and caregivers, in either the voluntary or proprietary sectors, are the typical sources for such devices and the training necessary to use them.

Adjunctive Health Services

Adjunctive health services include specialized activities such as occupational and physical therapy and speech and hearing interventions. They are essential to helping restore care recipients' adaptive capacities and preventing decline in functioning. Caregivers offer some of these services in formal settings such as clinics, hospitals, residential institutions, and day-care centers. They often occur in the home, where the vast majority of persons with disabilities live.

Emotional/Cognitive Resources

How we feel about ourselves and others, our attitude toward the world, the accuracy of our perceptions of reality, and our general ability to cope are among the features of our lives dependent on the availability of emotional/cognitive resources. As shown in table 4.1, services to provide these resources include support groups, counseling, and psychotherapy.

Support Groups

Peer-support groups have expanded over the past decade in large part because they meet a particular set of needs that are different from other services (Wuthnow 1994). We have placed this service under the category of emotional/cognitive, but it is clear that many informal caregivers want to interact with other informal caregivers to share their experiences in carrying out instrumental tasks associated with caregiving.

Through this sharing they learn firsthand from others who are involved in the day-to-day work of caregiving. Although professionals may have more theoretical or technical knowledge, informal caregivers often, through improvisation born of necessity, discover techniques of caregiving that have yet to become a part of the professionals' practice knowledge, and develop shortcuts to obtain needed community resources. Much of this mutual support activity occurs when informal caregivers and care recipients share their experiences informally in waiting rooms, schools, or community centers or talk at length by telephone. Professionals also conduct support groups for both care recipients and informal caregivers in many settings, including hospitals, community centers, schools, or treatment centers.

Professionals themselves need support. They experience criticism from patients and clients, family members, and other professionals and often feel that what they do makes little or no difference (see table 4.2). Being subject to these negative reactions, combined with feeling constantly overworked and not having sufficient time for personal or family life, means that formal caregivers must cope with much stress. Hay and Oken (1977) proposed the use of peer-support groups to help professionals cope with these and other stresses. Nottingham et al.'s (1993) finding that 94 percent of professionals saw linkage with other professionals to be very important also suggests the importance of such groups in providing emotional support. On the cognitive and skill side, they also permit sharing information about best practices. More than half of these formal caregivers reported that they did not have sufficient help in this area.

TABLE 4.2. Barriers to Caregiving

Personal Barriers	Relational Barriers	System Barriers	Cultural Barriers
Competing role demands: life events, family configuration	Aspects of caregiving role: frequency, timing, duration	Lack of coordination of services	Cultural/societal norms: resources
Personality: attitudes, beliefs, values	Aspects of relationship: history, quality	Availability: policies, insurance rules/regulations	Family history: resources
Physical health: age, energy	Relational characteristics: communication skills, negotiation skills, mutuality	Affordability: financial obligations, employment	Stigma related to caregiving and being cared for
Coping strategies		Accessibility: marketing strategies, geography, jargon and slang	
Intrapsychic strains		Lack of inter-/ intrapersonal training	

Counseling and Psychotherapy

The provision of social support is often an informal matter that occurs throughout daily life and applies to each of the transactions identified in table 4.1. In contrast, formal caregivers offer counseling and psychotherapy to care recipients, informal caregivers, and other professionals in organized service contexts. Counseling and psychotherapy are related, with psychotherapy tending to be a more specialized and pathology-oriented intervention requiring more advanced mental health training. They are often offered in conjunction with other services and can assist in making certain services, such as skilled medical care, more effective.

In an earlier part of this chapter, we discussed the different types of stress informal caregivers experience, some of which are caused by practical concerns and others because of intrapersonal and interpersonal concerns. Richmond (1973; Garrard and Richmond 1963) urged formal caregivers to attend to specific intrapersonal aspects of caregiving to improve services to the care recipient, while also helping the informal caregiver have a more successful and personally enriching role in the caregiving transaction. Specifically, Richmond (1973) described a process of adaptation that informal caregivers may undergo as they try to adapt to their caregiving roles. The specific aspects of this adaptation entail mechanisms of defense—denial, guilt, projection, and dependency—which often overlap in informal caregivers' attempts to come to grips with their demanding situation.

The process of *denial* may entail repeated requests for consultation with formal caregivers or for "second opinions" about the care recipients' illnesses. It may also take the form of an inability to share the problem with other potential informal caregivers, such as friends and family members. Regarding *guilt,* informal caregivers may blame themselves, for example, for not seeking medical care earlier in the course of care recipients' illnesses, which may result in depressive feelings. *Projection* occurs when informal caregivers blame others, such as formal caregivers or other family members, for care recipients' problems. Informal caregivers may also become too *dependent* on formal caregivers and agencies, on relatives, or even on the care recipient.

Recognizing informal caregivers' mechanisms of adaptation helps formal caregivers understand common processes they are likely to observe, how these processes may lead to certain informal caregiver behaviors, and how to manage the situation to maximize treatment efforts and the adaptation of all concerned. For example, formal caregivers may feel threatened when family members repeatedly ask questions and continue to misunderstand their responses, characteristic of the denial process. Again, formal caregivers may feel as if they are being attacked when informal caregivers blame them for care recipients' disorders, which often occurs as part of the projection mechanism. These transactions can develop into barriers to caring if formal caregivers do not recognize them as aspects of the adaptation process and if they do not handle them sensitively and effectively.

Summary and Conclusion

Table 4.1's overview of services and the material just presented suggest that all persons in caregiving transactions encounter common issues and stresses across diverse situations. Although the table seems to imply that the formal caregiver is the primary provider and the care recipient is the primary recipient, this is not the conclusion we want to draw. Although the professional caregivers are involved in a larger number of different types of services, informal caregivers actually provide more care when measured in volume and duration. The table suggests something often overlooked. The often unnoticed informal caregiver assumes great responsibility, has many needs, is susceptible to many stresses, and will become ever more important to the caregiving endeavor in the future. Thus, our belief is that plans for caregiving need to focus much more directly on the informal caregiver than has been the case and should address their needs through carefully and systematically designed services and policies.

In the previous section we identified a host of services organized into two categories: (1) those providing instrumental resources designed to meet immediate needs and make the caregiving task less burdensome, and (2) those providing emotional/cognitive resources designed to help persons in the caregiving situation cope better and to enhance the effectiveness of other services. These services can help reduce stressors causing considerable burdens to caregivers, reduce burnout, delay or prevent unnecessary institutionalization, and positively affect the quality of life of all involved in caregiving. Yet we know that even when these services are in place, people underutilize them, and they frequently lack effectiveness (Moroney 1977). Why? What are the barriers to service delivery and use?

We reviewed a range of work on barriers and identified a number of them (Avison et al. 1993; Biegel, Sales, and Schulz 1991; Freudenberger 1990; Goldfarb et al. 1986; Gray 1990; McPheeters 1990; Mullan 1993; Stephens 1993; Walker 1989). The following section begins to deal with some of these.

Issues of Communication and Culture

We use the term *communication* in a broader sense than is usually the case. Communication is more than just one person telling another person something, and it goes beyond reciprocal exchanges where people share information with each other. Rather, we use the term in the sense that Habermas uses it. In chapter 3 we introduced the notion of "communicative competency," a process of exchange that also involves the development of trust between those who are in dialogue. We discussed the meaning of such concepts as truth, legitimacy, sincerity, and clarity and the foundation for building a trusting relationship. We suggested further that people who are "competent" in their ability to "communicate" with others are people who are capable of building a relationship that meets Schön's definition of Model II practice.

And yet, we argue that many of the informal caregivers we have described in this chapter, who are experiencing stress and who would benefit from services, are not receiving them even when they are available in their communities. To a large extent, it is because the professional caregiver has certain expectations that are grounded in Model I behavior, expectations that often are different from the informal caregiver. These attitudes and their resulting behaviors stand in the way of any meaningful partnership.

To achieve this partnership, the professional needs to go beyond the rhetoric and more fully understand that

∾ informal caregivers are, for the most part, capable caregivers;

∾ informal caregivers should be an integral part of the service delivery team and should be part of the decision-making process as it affects the care recipient;

∾ informal caregivers experience considerable stress in their roles as caregivers;

∾ most informal caregivers will benefit if provided supportive services; and

∾ some informal caregivers will themselves experience problems because of the demands of caregiving and will need treatment services themselves.

If the above is to be realized, informal caregivers need to be recognized as the essential and primary providers of care. It is they, not the professionals, who have assumed the responsibility for the care recipient.

Professionals should expect family members, relatives, and friends to behave like informal caregivers, not like professionals. Since they have assumed the responsibility and burden of providing care, their efforts should be supported by the professional, who needs to demonstrate trust in and respect for their decisions, their styles, and their efforts.

The reality is far from the ideal.

∾ A large number of professionals tend to view informal caregivers as potential barriers to the care recipient's successful treatment.

∾ Others see the informal caregivers as extensions of the professional or the professional team. While the professional maintains overall responsibility for treatment, he or she does delegate some tasks to the informal caregiver, who will carry them out under the supervision of the professional.

∾ A significantly smaller number of professionals recognize the informal caregivers as the primary caregivers and define their tasks as supportive.

The first two views, instead of promoting the involvement of the informal caregiver, discourage their participation in a meaningful manner. First, although there might be lip service for their participation, the actual participation is usually marginal. Second, professionals typically maintain their expert role and discount the knowledge, experiences, and abilities of the informal caregivers. Even though they may have heard what the informal caregiver said, they did not value it or incorporate it into their thinking about the situation. This approach fosters dependence instead of promoting empowerment and interdependency. The third view is clearly supportive to informal caregivers in the sense that they are seen as capable caregivers if they are supported.

If professionals are to move beyond an intellectual acceptance of the principles underpinning the third view, they have to realize that the cultural context in which caregiving relationships evolve is based in norms, values, beliefs, and practices that influence decisions and actions that may not be helpful or harmful to the informal caregiver or the care recipient. We believe, like Matthews (1993), that the specific factors that become barriers are cultural norms, community resources, and historical content of family traditions. Mullan (1993) included the lack of social support from friends or family as a barrier when the failure is based on attitudes and beliefs. Informal caregivers will choose not to seek needed professional help if there is criticism from significant others when help is sought (Stephens 1993). Such criticism yields the stigma that informal caregivers and those they are caring for fear will be attached to them in their caregiving relationships.

The barrier created by fear of being stigmatized can be a major problem that tends to have multiplicative effects. For example, the care recipient who does not seek help because of a fear that she or he will be perceived as weak and dependent may delay until the condition progresses to the point where the treatment is less likely to have an effect. Parents of children with disabilities sometimes choose not to seek formal services because of fear of being stigmatized by friends, family, or the community (Goldfarb et al. 1986). This problem easily leads to caregiving burnout. Thus, cultural barriers can affect the caregiver/care recipient transactions such that those needing formal help do not seek it. The following account of one informal caregiver's experience illustrates how damaging the cultural stigma can be:

> When my husband first started showing signs of mental illness, all of our family and friends were truly supportive. Many of our friends referred to his problems as a "nervous breakdown" and lumped my husband into the list of other friends who had suffered nervous breakdowns. Then, when this "breakdown" progressed and was diagnosed as a more permanent mental disorder, we lost our friends; even family members began to make excuses for not visiting. It was difficult for me to get respite, because at first there was no one to help, then, later, I began to feel embarrassed about the whole situation.

Cultural barriers result from the stereotypes of the professional world that many people hold. Goldfarb et al. (1986) report that informal caregivers tend to shy away from developing a formal support system among themselves because of attitudes of professionals. Walker (1989) documented examples of how parents' stereotypes of the formal system prevented them from establishing formal support for getting services for their children with disabilities. Many times it is the attitudes and attributions that informal caregivers and care recipients have of the formal system that serve as barriers to taking initiative and seeking services.

Cross (1989), in her foundational publication *Towards a Culturally Competent System of Care*, offers a thoughtful and detailed discussion of what culturally competent practice would entail. She offers the following principles as a beginning point for such an approach. Culturally competent practice begins with a commitment on the part of the professional (1) to acknowledge that culture is a predominant force in shaping behaviors, values, and institutions and that the family provides the context within which these are internalized by individual members; and (2) to acknowledge cultural differences and the ways in which these differences affect the helping process. Within this context, the professional needs to accept that each culture finds some behaviors, interactions, or values more important than others; these are found in communication patterns, life view, and definitions of health and well-being. Following this, (3) the professional needs to develop a dual perspective by first understanding the role of culture in one's own life and being aware of one's own ethnocentricism and then making a conscious effort to understand the meaning of a caregiver's or care recipient's behavior within his or her cultural context, especially help-seeking behavior.

Given this, the professional caregiver should be able to begin a helping relationship with an openness to learn from the informal caregiver what is considered "normal" in their informal culture and what to expect in terms of behaviors typical of an encounter with a professional; adapt practices that accommodate what the informal caregiver expects in terms of social decorum and etiquette; adapt interviewing styles to accommodate the informal caregiver's communication pattern that is influenced by his or her culture.

The Development of Caring

As we noted in chapter 1, caring is a quality of the caregiving relationship that develops through communication. It is based on a commitment of the caregiver to the well-being of the care recipient with an attitude of respect and dignity. It, like all affective bonds, may not be as strong at the beginning as later, or vice versa, depending on the way the transactions work out. Caring is the ideal of the I-Thou relationship (Buber 1958). Ideally, the caring relationship would be mutual: both parties would share dignity and respect for each other and "work" for the personal development of the other. Unhappily, that is unlikely. Often the care recipient is unable to reciprocate, and the relationship is one-sided. It is necessary, therefore, to expand our thinking about who is in the caregiving transaction and include someone else.

For example, in chapter 3, we saw that the caregiving relationship can be markedly improved by the addition of additional formal and informal caregivers. It expands the possibilities that all involved can engage in a respectful relationship with someone in the system. Mutually supportive caregiving can then happen in a "microcommunity" social grouping, where at least some of the participants are familiar with Model II approaches and can help the others develop that way of functioning. The goal is of communicative competence of all parties.

5 ❧   Caring about the Caregiver: Implications for the Organization and Delivery of Services

IN THE PREVIOUS CHAPTER, we argued that many caregivers find it difficult to provide the care required by their relatives, friends, and neighbors. This is affected in part by the kind of care they are called on to give and the intensity of the caregiving. In time, caregivers find themselves experiencing stress that threatens the relationship they have with the care receiver. We then identified the types of services that, if provided by the formal caregiving system, would ease this stress and restore some sense of equilibrium into the situation. Finally, we suggested that a major barrier to the caregivers being able to obtain these services often is found in the attitudes, behaviors, and practices of the professional caregivers.

Although these barriers might be surmounted if professionals would move toward a practice grounded in a reflective model (Model II), we recognize that professional practice is also influenced by the systems and organizations in which the professional operates. No matter how much the professional might want to change the nature of his or her practice, the extent to which this is possible is influenced by the availability of resources as well as administrative, operating fiscal, and legal policies and procedures. This chapter identifies, discusses, and critiques this second set of barriers.

The Issue of Resource Constraints

Despite the considerable growth in social welfare expenditures over the past thirty years, there are still significant shortages, and these shortages are continuing to be felt by informal caregivers who are carrying the major responsibility for the care of so many family members, relatives, and friends. Although these caregivers may be in a better position than their counterparts of the 1940s and 1950s in that few community-based services existed then or were in their infancy, these caregivers are still considered "less needy" than other at-risk groups.

In fact, the rhetoric of today, shaped by a perception of an economy in danger because of uncontrollable public spending, is to limit, at least for the time being, health and social services to those with the most acute and pressing need: children at risk of ill treatment, the very old and severely handicapped living alone, the mentally ill and mentally retarded in urgent need of care, and families at imminent risk of breakdown.

It is somewhat simplistic to assume that once the current economic "crisis" is reversed and the country enters into another expansionary period, resources will be plentiful enough so that such social services will be available to informal caregivers. Such a rationale suggests that their needs can only be met when there is a surplus of funds. This becomes problematic given the projections offered in chapter 2. We anticipate a growing number of elderly who will not be able to care for themselves and who do not have family members, relatives, or friends available or willing to provide that care. We anticipate a growing number of physically handicapped or emotionally disturbed children who also will need the formal caregiving system to substitute for family members who are unwilling or unable to provide for them.

Given this, current estimates of need must be treated with caution. In fact, there is every likelihood that once a targeted level of provision has been achieved, new demand will have been generated, and targets will have to be adjusted upward. The critical issue is not that the adjustments will have to be made but rather that, in establishing new priorities, informal caregivers will find themselves in no better position than they were before.

There are other limitations to an approach based on supply, demand, and needs analysis. Guidelines for service provision are rarely proposed as a set plan of action; but once developed, these guidelines have a tendency to become the detailed operational blueprint. The estimates become set in stone, and the ensuing programs often become ends in themselves rather than instruments to achieve some objectives. They generate their own dynamism, and over time they can reduce any efforts to initiate change through more flexible experimentation as the major concern of the administrators is for organizational survival.

Those responsible for the management of programs tend to structure their agencies in such a way that the purpose of the organization is defined as the sum total of their service components. Supervisors and front-line professionals find themselves viewing potential clients in terms of what services they are in a position to offer rather than what the caregiver or care recipient might actually need. Needs are translated invariably into what a particular agency has to offer. Although this is an overstatement, as a pattern it is commonly found in most bureaucracies. Flexibility may exist, but it is usually limited to a successful manipulation of the existing service package (Kettner, Moroney, and Martin 1990).

For any number of reasons, services that were introduced initially as possible mechanisms to assist people with needs quickly become *the* way to do things. Services that were seen as potentially beneficial become solutions whose benefit is rarely questioned. Innovation is replaced with caution, and flexibility with formal structures.

And yet, it is impossible to compartmentalize neatly the needs of informal caregivers. Moreover, it is critical that professionals understand that not only do needs differ among caregivers but a particular caregiver's needs will change over time. We need to develop mechanisms that build on the key notion of *choice.* Many family members have made a choice to become caregivers rather than transferring this function to the formal caregiving system, a nursing home, or other long-term care institution. Choice, of course, is not a simple concept—nor can it be limited to an either-or situation—and suggesting that informal caregivers have such a choice in no way implies that either course (informal or formal caregiving system) is equally desirable in all cases or that both serve the same function. The choice is meaningful only when there is a range of alternatives from which to choose. If the informal caregiver turns to the formal system, that system should offer choices from an array of services (both institutional and community based) that are of the highest quality. Choice also implies that the informal caregiver is viewed as carrying major responsibility for the decision and that professionals should not impose one course of action over another even if they believe it to be more appropriate.

Building on the principle of "shared responsibility," choice, real choice, implies a diversity of options, flexible enough to meet the needs of the informal caregiver and available when required. It would involve the development and provision of a wide range of alternative health and social services (basically those discussed in the previous chapter), and these services need to be offered as supports to caregivers and not, as we find in practice, services that substitute for the caregiver.

The challenge, then, is not only to develop and provide these services but also to create systems that foster flexibility, creativity, choice, and responsiveness.

Systemic Barriers

The development of such a system needs to confront four major problems: fragmentation, inaccessibility, discontinuity, and lack of accountability mechanisms.

Fragmentation of Services

Fragmentation refers to the problems associated with specialization, duplication of services, and the lack of cooperation among service providers (Agranoff 1977). A fragmented service delivery system creates a number of serious problems for caregivers and care recipients, but this "problem" historically was the solution to a previous problem. As we learned more about various conditions and problems, we found that the early-twentieth-century notion of a generalist, whether he or she was a physician, a social worker, a nurse, or other human service professional, was no longer viable. No one person could keep abreast of the new knowledge that was being generated. Professional education began to emphasize the training of specialists, and graduates identified themselves as experts in more narrow fields of practice. This evolution had numerous benefits to the patient or client whose specific problem was dealt with by a specialist in that area.

This same evolution was mirrored in the development of organizations and institutions in which these specialists worked. In many cases, services were organized by disease category (for example, heart disease, cancer, mental disabilities), by specific functions (such as vocational rehabilitation or meals on wheels), or by professional discipline (for instance, public health nurses, family and marital counseling).

Although specialization solved the problem of an exploding knowledge base, resulting in better outcomes in resolving specific problems, specialization created a new set of problems. Most of the people who needed help had more than one need or problem, and these needs rarely fitted neatly into the service mix of a single agency. The problem was more than just one of caregivers or care recipients having to go from professional to professional, from agency to agency to have all their needs met. More often than not, they never got to these other providers or did so after considerable delay. Each professional, expert in his or her own practice, was often the victim of a form of "professional myopia." They neither recognized nor looked for these other problems, and the caregiver or care recipient was limited to the specific services of the particular professional. Said one informal caregiver:

> I care for my mentally ill sister and two other mentally ill people, who are not relatives, in my home. All three of them must go regularly to the same two clinics for appointments. Not only will the clinics not send someone to my home to conduct the meetings, they usually say they are unable to schedule the meetings at a common time. This means that I have to take these three ladies to two different clinics, in different parts of town, on three different days, for six different appointments; this makes six trips, rather than two trips. It would surely be easier for me and the three ladies to either have coordinated meetings, or for a caseworker to come to our home; but, I also think it would be more efficient for them.

Inaccessibility of Services

Even when services are available in their community, caregivers and care recipients find themselves victimized by another set of barriers that effectively keep them from obtaining these services. These barriers include the caregivers' not knowing that the services actually exist, or, even if they do know of them, being excluded because of restrictive eligibility policies (Agranoff 1977).

Caserta et al. (1987) found that almost half of the informal caregivers surveyed in their study reported that they did not know of formal community services available in their areas, even though they were part of support groups at the time of the surveys. Stephens (1993) suggested that lack of knowledge of services is among the main reasons why formal services are not used, citing a study by the Office of Technology Assessment (1988).

As an example, the following account exemplifies how a lack of knowledge about a specific disorder, potentially a result of inaccessible services, served as a barrier to a daughter caring for her father:

> The main problem is with my father's sight, and I don't know anything about visual impairments—so many things that I did not know that would have made it so much easier for my father. For example, I didn't know that I should let him hold onto me; I didn't know to tell him how many steps there were between rooms, I didn't know how to explain to him where his food was on his plate. If I had known that people with visual impairments often like to see bright colors, or might like to listen to music or birds singing, I would have done this for him. It would have made such a difference to have known more about this.

The potential for legal issues to become substantial barriers to caregiving is great when one considers the process of obtaining treatment for someone suffering from a mental illness. When the courts convene to determine whether he or she needs involuntary treatment, they often do this by judging whether the person is "dangerous to him- or herself, or to others," which generally depends on whether someone has witnessed their attempt to commit suicide or whether family members, relatives, or friends have been threatened with bodily harm by the care recipient. Even though the law was originally developed to encourage treatment, some are denied treatment because they do not appear to be dangerous to themselves or others (Burland 1992). This same problem exists in situations when parents are caring for severely emotionally disturbed children. Services are expensive, and most insurance plans offer limited assistance, forcing parents reluctantly to declare in court that they are "unwilling" to continue providing care. They are forced to request that the court, through the state's child welfare system, take over parental responsibility. The ability to pay for services is another concern to caregivers; in addition, in a number of communities, caregivers who can pay find that many needed services are funded by Title XX (the Social Services Block Grant) and are restricted to those whose income and resources are below the poverty level.

Discontinuity of Services

Discontinuity refers to the lack of communication and joint efforts between and among providers (Agranoff 1977). For a service delivery plan to be responsive, it must identify not only the various services needed but also when each service will be delivered. Providers often do not coordinate among themselves but expect care recipients or informal caregivers to serve as their own service coordinators. As discussed under the issue of "fragmentation," they must often rely on several different professional caregivers to provide them with an array of needed services. When the professional does not take responsibility for helping the care recipient and caregiver to navigate the system, two major problems can arise. First, most nonprofessionals are unable to deal with the logistics of organizing the type of complete service plan many of their children, parents, relatives, or friends need. They have neither the expertise nor the time that is required. Beyond the often impossible task of organizing services from various providers, caregivers are faced with the equally problematic responsibility of informing each professional of their needs and how they as a provider fit into a larger picture.

This issue was commented on by a number of respondents in the survey conducted by the Rosalynn Carter Institute. They experienced a lack of cooperation from professionals, and they believed that professionals were bound by various rules and regulations; they also believed professionals felt a lack of administrative support that could potentially lead to a drain on the professionals' creativity, motivation, and incentive in dealing with their situations.

Lack of Accountability

This barrier is created when there is "a lack of interactive relationships between the individuals being served and the organizations' decision makers, such as inability of clients to influence decisions that affect them or the insensitivity of service providers to clients' needs and interests" (Agranoff 1977, 531). There are a number of issues involved in this: (1) a lack of a mechanism that allows a care recipient or caregiver to question and hold accountable specific providers when they feel that they are not being treated fairly and appropriately; (2) a lack of a system that identifies the need for monitoring the quality of services across the community; and (3) a lack of a systemwide oversight function that brings agency personnel, boards of directors, consumers, and advocates together to plan and to evaluate services.

Proposed Solutions

Services Integration

Eliot Richardson (1973), a former secretary of health, education, and welfare (now health and human services), addressed these barriers when he argued for

> developing an integrated framework within which ongoing programs can be rationalized and enriched to do a better job of making services available within existing commitments and resources. Its objectives must include such things as (1) the coordinated delivery of services for the greatest benefit of the people, (2) a holistic approach to the individual and the family unit, (3) the provision of a comprehensive range of services locally, (4) the rational allocation of resources at the local level so as to be responsive to local needs. (2)

Taking its lead from Richardson's charge, the service integration movement of the late 1960s and the 1970s implemented a number of projects that had many elements in common. First, at the policy level, mechanisms were established that (1) emphasized the need to provide consumer-based, agency-neutral assessments of need; (2) suggested mechanisms to establish priorities and allocate resources that were in the best interest of the consumer rather than continuing a process that was controlled by the agencies; (3) required an evaluation system that measured systemwide outcomes; and (4) recommended a governance structure that established working procedures between agencies. The new emphasis was on creating and strengthening the *system* rather than on individual providers. Early service integration efforts were a major part of the War on Poverty—Community Action Agencies, the Model Cities Programs, the A-95 federal grant review process at the federal level, and the numerous initiatives at the state level to reorganize government through the creation of "umbrella" departments combining agencies such as health, mental health, social services, vocational rehabilitation, and others.

While the above are examples of efforts to meet the policy and programmatic concerns we have been discussing, related activities were being implemented at the micro level. These included the development of centralized intake capabilities, information and referral services, and, possibly the most important innovation, the introduction of case management.

As discussed earlier in this chapter, if professionals are to be more responsive to the needs of informal caregivers, they must know how to be more "holistic" in their approach; that is, they must be more informed about the potential multiple needs of their clients (for example, health, vocational training, income support, mental health, family counseling, legal, personal care), the availability of services to meet the multiple needs, and how they can link their clients to other service providers.

Since most professionals will need to continue to be specialists in their respective disciplines, they cannot, at the same time, be experts in these additional areas. Still they will need some awareness of these needs and services if they are to function well within an integrated services framework. One of the continuing challenges will be that of balancing the need for professionals with specialized and highly technical knowledge and skills with the need for generalist professionals and informal caregivers who can negotiate bureaucratic hurdles and fragmented services (Stephens 1993; Caserta et al. 1987).

Most services integration models have utilized the function of a *service coordinator* (or *case manager*). The success of this "generalist" depends on his or her (a) ability to carry out comprehensive client needs assessments, (b) working knowledge of the human service system, (c) ability to link clients with the appropriate agency or professional practitioner, (d) ability to function as an effective client advocate, and (e) ability to monitor the experience of the client as he or she is provided services by these agencies and practitioners.

If service integration is to be realized, professionals must learn to become collaborative members of service teams. Efforts to coordinate services involve not just the sharing of space (that is, co-location of offices) but also the sharing of common databases about clients and services, developing common intake forms, consolidating business support operations (for example, billing, personnel, marketing), joint planning of services, and negotiating responsibility for how acceptable outcomes of services will be defined. In effect, professionals will need to practice more in the mode of Schön's reflective practitioner than has been traditionally the case.

Parallel to the service integration movement was the emergence during the late 1970s and early 1980s of family-support programs. A major stimulus was the formation of the Family Resource Coalition—consisting of more than three hundred programs—in 1981. As reported in *America's Family Support Programs* (Kagan et al. 1987), these programs were found in school settings, social service agencies, child care agencies, corporations, and hospitals.

> Family support programs reflect the ecological orientation in that they mediate between the family and more remote and bureaucratized institutions such as corporations and government agencies. In some cases, programs help families navigate complex systems to obtain basic services. In other cases, via support programs, families may mobilize to advocate for improved services or for changes in bureaucratic policies. (Kagan et al. 1987, 10)

As discussed throughout this book, family members as informal caregivers provide a significant amount of the services and supports required by care recipients. When care recipients also require the services of professionals, family members must become active participants in the advocacy for and planning and provision of services. This was the major agenda of the family-support programs—the blending of the provision of direct services and advocacy: "By direct service we mean the educative and supportive events and activities offered by programs that help individuals (and families). By advocacy we mean activities that seek to propel changes in organizational practice or in governmental or institutional policy" (Kagan et al. 1987, 366).

A more recent review of family-support programs in fourteen local communities can be found in *Family Investment Strategies: Improving the Lives of Children and Communities* (Pines 1994).

Emerging from these efforts is the recognition that professionals need to look more carefully at the assets and resources that family members and care recipients can bring to caregiving transactions. While there is still a consideration of illness and disability, there is a growing focus on strength and ability and the personal and material resources that can be applied in caregiving situations.

Human services are in the process of shifting to more integrated, holistic approaches to care recipients and their informal caregivers. Formal caregivers are adjusting to the sharing of responsibility and decision making with care recipients and informal caregivers. Services are increasingly emphasizing community-based, noninstitutional interventions with more and more attention to preventing or postponing illness and promoting healthy lifestyle choices. There is a correlated shift taking place away from pathology-based models and toward wellness models. Increasingly, all parties in caregiving transactions are evaluating services in terms of client outcomes and less in terms of provider and system inputs.

Other developments have been occurring that affect, not so much the structure of services, but rather the manner in which services are delivered and the way in which professionals have been required to adjust their approaches to their practice. The following discussion reviews some of these delivery system developments. Furthermore, although none of these innovations emphasized the needs of informal caregivers, our analysis and critique of each strategy focuses on whether they are achieving their stated objectives. Following this we discuss whether these programs are potentially of benefit, are neutral toward, or actually penalize these caregivers.

Block Grants

Historically, the federal government has utilized the politically expedient grants-in-aid approach to meet the social and health needs of people. This pattern supports the strong historical preference for state and local administration of domestic programs. While some benefits such as Social Security and other income transfer programs are provided by the federal government directly, the great bulk of public services in health, education, housing, highway construction, and parks and recreation are provided by state and local governments with partial funding from the federal government.

Federal participation has, of course, increased significantly throughout the twentieth century. By the 1920s and into the 1930s, federal grants-in-aid were available for vocational education, vocational rehabilitation, and maternal and child health programs. During the depression, a dozen major grant programs were enacted. These were justified with the argument that the resources of state and local governments were inadequate since they were unable to raise sufficient revenues. Furthermore, it was argued that not only were state and local taxes inflexible and regressive but also citizens would not receive equal treatment, since some states were poorer than others and still others developed discriminatory policies that led to the withholding of services to various groups of people based on their race or ethnicity.

These grants-in-aid programs, also referred to as categorical programs, established national goals, goals that transcended the right of state and local governments to decide on what services should be provided. National goals implied that citizens had rights that only the federal government could guarantee. Through these programs, the federal government in effect told the states that they would receive federal funds but could only use them for specific types of programs. In fact, the federal government required that the states establish mandated organizational structures, deliver prescribed services, and accept certain federally determined eligibility standards.

The creation of those programs did effectively deal with the specific problems of targeted populations, but the later movement toward block grants may be seen as a reaction to some of the problems created by categorical funding—that is, as they evolved, they were no longer person-focused, individualistic, or flexible but rather program-focused, rule-driven, rigid, and not coordinated with other services.

Beginning in the mid-1960s, a number of block grants were developed in housing and community development. While cities were given these funds to combat urban problems (in this sense they were still categorical), they were also given considerable latitude in how they were to spend the money. In the early 1970s Title XX of the Social Security Act was passed, and block grants moved from the status of demonstration and experimentation to that of preferred federal government policy.

In the 1980s, the federal government expanded the block grant programs. Categorical programs increasingly gave way to this new approach. These included major block grants in the area of mental health and social services. In the 1990s, Congress has proposed an even greater expansion of block grants in the areas of child welfare, welfare reform, and medical care.

While states are offered these funds with fewer strings attached than under previous categorical programs, the federal government also imposed ceilings on their share of the financing. The goal of greater state control of how the funds were to be spent has been tempered with the equally important federal goal of cost containment.

Additional Reform Proposals

In their book *Reinventing Government,* Osborne and Gaebler (1992) discuss the advantages of market-oriented government as involving the changing of systems (government services, competition, customer choice, accountability for results, and public enterprise). They note, however, that markets can create inequitable outcomes (for example, poor people with limited access to health care). Because of this, Osborne and Gaebler stress the need to improve communities: "To complement the efficiency and effectiveness of market mechanisms, we need the warmth and caring of families and neighborhoods and communities. As entrepreneurial governments move away from administrative bureaucracies, they need to embrace both markets *and* community" (309).

Two significant attempts to move in this direction are the growth of *purchase of service contracting (POSC)* and *managed care.* The federal government first authorized state welfare departments to purchase services from other state agencies through amendments to the Social Security Act passed in 1962. In this early attempt in welfare reform, the federal government not only encouraged states to purchase services from other agencies but also increased their match for social services from 50 percent to 75 percent; left social services open ended; and significantly expanded the eligible population. Through the 1967 amendments to the Social Security Act, Congress encouraged the states not only to expand purchase of service contracting but to purchase these services from private agencies.

Thirty years later, purchase of service contracting has expanded and has also become the preferred vehicle for financing many of the human services to the point that most private, not-for-profit agencies are dependent on these contracts for their survival (Eggers and Ng 1993; McMurtry et al. 1990). Under this program, agencies agree to provide a specific number of units of services to designated client populations. State agencies, beyond deciding on what services are to be delivered to whom, have the responsibility to monitor the contracts, that is, they are concerned that the services are actually delivered and that they meet established quality standards. However, little, if any, attention to date has been given to evaluating the effectiveness of these services as to whether recipients are better off because of the services they received.

At the same time that the private agencies came to depend more heavily on these contracts, Congress began to cut back on the amount of federal dollars allocated for these services—as part of the block grant strategy; the new partnership was driven by what has become known as the "block, cap, and cut" approach to human services.

Kettner and Martin (1996), in their assessment of the impact of POSC on the private sector, found in their sample of ninety-eight agencies drawn from all fifty states that, while 82 percent of the agencies reported that demand was increasing from clients who could not pay anything toward the costs of the services and more than 90 percent of the agencies reported that demand was increasing from clients who could pay something but not all of the costs of the services, 45 percent of the agencies were forced to accept fewer clients, more clients were placed on waiting lists, 63 percent were forced to increase staff workloads, and 42 percent had to terminate programs in light of reduced funding.

Kettner and Martin (1996) also cite the findings of Knapp et al. (1990) suggesting that POSC has the potential for "fragmentation, discontinuity, complexity, low quality outputs, poorly targeted services, productive inefficiencies, and inappropriate replication, sectarianism and paternalism" (24) and Gronbjerg (1990), who found that "private, nonprofit agencies devote most of their efforts to serving middle and upper-middle income groups" (24).

Managed care is a more recent innovation in the human services field, emerging in the 1980s. Unlike block grants and purchase of service contracting, which on one level offer more responsibility and flexibility to the states to determine what services will be offered and allow for new partnerships between the public and private sectors while on another level have been the major instruments of cutbacks in the amount of resources available to the states, managed care has turned the human service system around, especially in the health and mental health fields. Flexibility has given way to a highly structured and rigid set of policies and procedures that determine the type and amount of services that providers will be allowed to deliver. Managed care is basically concerned with cost containment, and the organizations that reimburse providers are in a position to determine how much they will pay.

Professional judgment and discretion have been diminished to the point where the needs of clients are only a part of the decision-making calculus. The concept of allowable costs has become more significant in determining what will be done. Although this concept is different in many ways from the strategy of using Diagnostic Related Groupings (DRGs) introduced in the mid-1980s, one similarity is their reliance on relating the provision of services to a predetermined idea of what a typical client with a typical problem (diagnosis) will need. Furthermore, if providers exceed this level of services, the third-party payer will not reimburse them for these "additional" services.

Finally, the federal government, through the Government Performance and Results Act of 1993 (P.L. 103–61) and the administration's proposed Performance Act, will require government at all levels to establish *performance measures* for all federally funded programs falling under what will be known as Performance Partnership Grants (PPGs). While the operationalization of this new emphasis is still being worked out, some elements are taking shape, especially in the area of the process to be used to determine acceptable performance measurements.

The performance measurement movement is proposed as a management tool, not to be used to determine cutbacks and contain costs as its primary goal, but to "clarify what we want to achieve, document the contribution that we can make to achieving our goals, and document what we are getting for our investment" (DHHS 1995, 19).

To develop these measures, "important stakeholders, . . . from organizations representing potential grant recipients . . . selected not only for their personal expertise or perspective, but also because they have shown an ability to foster participation by interested stakeholders who are not able to attend the meetings" (DHHS 1995, 19), will be asked, in advance of the meetings, to indicate what results they would identify as important to their individual programs. This information, in turn, will be the basis for discussions at the regional meetings. The output from the regional meetings—lists of desired program results—will then be reviewed by various federal agencies that will evaluate them from a technical perspective (for example, are they measurable, are they feasible).

The third phase of the process involves asking those who participated in the regional meetings to comment on the technical report and make additional recommendations to the Department of Health and Human Services. Phases Four and Five involve the development of operational state plans to achieve the agreed-upon objectives and the actualization of meaningful partnerships among the affected stakeholders.

We have included this program even though it is still evolving because it is likely to be widely implemented and, more important, because the program will probably have significant effects on informal caregivers.

Implications of These Developments
for Informal Caregivers

Few disagree with the ideas and philosophy underpinning service integration, but many professionals are uncomfortable with the actual implementation of such a system. Although such a system should produce cost savings over time, start-up costs can be high, and in times of shrinking resources, providers often find it difficult to divert scarce funds from service delivery to organizational restructuring. Moreover, many professionals believe that service integration will result in a loss of either their individual or their agency's autonomy—fears that are real. If the efforts to develop these mechanisms do not also include a recognition of these realities, and if efforts do not include the building of trust within the various parts of the system, the development of a responsive service integration system will be impossible.

There are considerable technical challenges involved in the achievement of the above tasks, but it is important to recognize that there has also been an underlying struggle for control involved, that is, between proponents of service integration and those who are concerned with strengthening the specialized agencies and providers. For these advocates of the existing fragmented system, service integration would result in a lowering of quality and a lessening of individual autonomy.

The challenge to the proponents of integrated services is to convince special-interest advocates that the integration of services will not result in a diminution of services or fewer resources for them. They also need to convince the special-interest advocates that the integration and consolidation of services will result in such efficiencies of operation that additional funding will then be made available for direct services to clients. To date, this challenge has not been met. While there are some examples of service integration projects still in operation, and while there is evidence that they have successfully dealt with the problems of fragmentation, accessibility, lack of accountability, poor communication, and lack of cooperation among providers, these efforts are limited.

Block grants pose a different set of problems. Some of the proponents of integrated services have expressed alarm that the expansion of block grants will adversely affect certain populations. Part of the alarm has stemmed from concern that block grants would make it difficult for advocates to identify where either the Congress or state legislatures reduced funds previously available. Part has stemmed from the same concern that originally motivated the proponents of categorical funding, that is, that without specifying by category (of disease, population, or service) the intended use of appropriated funds, one's favorite cause would suffer.

Purchase of service contracting and managed care are likely to have a negative effect on informal caregivers. Throughout this book we have emphasized that, given the nature of the caregiving process most family members, relatives, and friends are involved in, the formal system must make services available that begin with the notion of choice and are not only flexible but packaged creatively.

It is one thing to provide services to those who do not have family members available or willing to assist in the caring process; it is much more difficult to plan for those situations where the handicapped person is living with his or her family, where the family has assumed the major caring responsibility. First, the focus has shifted from the care recipient, a shift that is more significant than may appear on the surface. The task is no longer one of assessing an individual's capacity to function and then to provide services that substitute for the family. What is required now is the provision of services that ease the management task of the family. If policy planning requires an ability to categorize needs and then a capability to aggregate these needs, the process logically begins with a search for similarities between individuals rather than their differences.

This search for common needs becomes quite difficult when we realize that these caregivers have needs that vary widely. Furthermore, flexibility in the provision of services is often antithetical to the needs of planners as they attempt to structure services. The categories are not neatly defined.

Purchase of service contracting and managed care emphasize commonalities rather than differences. The former has strengthened the existing and traditional service delivery system, and contracts are often given to agencies to provide what they have always provided. The latter, on the other hand, is built on the notion that it is possible to determine what type of services and how many units of those services the average client with an average diagnosis needs. The value of diversity and individual need has given way to the value of offering services based on the notion of the lowest common denominator.

Finally, we pointed out early in this chapter that as resources become scarcer, the ensuing process to establish priorities will push many families further back in the queue. Block grants, purchase of service contracting, and managed care are the major policy instruments to achieve the perceived cuts in human service outlays.

The final and most recent innovation—performance measurement—while still untested, has the potential of benefiting informal caregivers. It allows for an open process so that various "stakeholders" might come together and through a structured dialogue inform each other and eventually establish priorities. Moreover, the process appears to be concerned not so much with cost cutting as with funding those programs with the potential for achieving important outcomes for the consumers of those programs and producing benefits for the larger society.

The one caveat we have is that the process of identifying and involving appropriate participants in this dialogue is unclear. Informal caregivers as such are not organized. At best they are found in a number of formal organizations, but these organizations are likely to advocate *not* for informal caregivers as such but for the needs of the patients, clients, or consumers of these organizations. To ensure that their needs will be included in the agenda, informal caregivers will need to come together in an organization that focuses on their needs rather than on the needs of those to whom they are providing care. Can they do this without assistance, or is it likely that such an effort is only possible through a new partnership with professional caregivers and concerned agencies?

6 ∾   Caring for the Caregivers: An Agenda

In PREVIOUS CHAPTERS, we discussed the importance of professionals understanding with greater sensitivity the amount of caregiving, usually at great personal and interpersonal costs, that informal caregivers are providing. This chapter explores two major themes that have emerged as critical if we are to develop responsive services to support caregivers. The first is concerned with the training of the helping professionals, the second with the empowerment of informal caregivers. Although other issues are important, we believe that these two are essential if partnerships are to be realized and integrated services achieved.

Professional Training

Three groups of professionals are key to achieving the goals of partnership (Twigg 1992). By "key" we do not intend to imply that others such as psychologists, counselors, and therapists are not important resources. Rather, we need to recognize that (1) there are a limited number of these professionals compared with the number of primary physicians, nurses, and social workers, and (2) they are not usually in front-line positions interacting with clients when the problem/need arises. More often than not, they function at the second level: specialized resources to whom the others refer patients. The first key professional is the "family doctor" or the general practitioner. Historically, this is the person with whom most caregivers and care recipients have contact. Given this, they are in a position to assess the total needs of the family, mobilize resources, and serve as an advocate when necessary.

Unfortunately, general practitioners are not trained to deal with the social aspects of patient care, and unless they make home visits, they are often unaware of the impact of caring on the informal caregiver. Practice is usually limited to the office visit, a contact that is time-limited given the demands on the physician's time, the economics of practice, and the inevitability of large-scale managed care initiatives. Finally, most general practitioners are unprepared to deal with the issue of community resources. They are not trained to do so, nor is the structure of practice supportive. They have been socialized to function as individuals (or in group practice with other physicians) and have little contact with other human service professionals.

> General practitioners often lack any formal training in relation to the social dimensions of their work. As a result they tend to either avoid responding in these areas, or do so on the basis of "common sense" assumptions deriving from their own social worlds. . . . [Their] expectations of being in command make it difficult for them to refer to services over which they have no direct control. . . . As a result they prefer to refer to services in the health sector . . . [while carers'] needs tend to be in the social rather than the health sphere. (Twigg 1992, 73)

The second key professional is the community or public health nurse. These professionals are in a position to be a major resource to the caregiver. Their training in this specialty is more holistic than that of hospital or clinic nurses, with a major emphasis given to the social aspects of care. The nature of their practice tends to be interdisciplinary so that as a member of a team they have access to more information on community resources. More often than not, their base of practice is in the home rather than the office or hospital. Given this, they are able to observe caregivers and care recipients in "natural" settings rather than merely asking them about their experiences. Community nurses can provide information and advice on many of the instrumental needs as discussed in chapter 4. "Nurses are relevant to a range of problems faced by carers. In addition to skilled nursing input, they can give advice and help about the course and management of medical conditions; they can help with incontinence and bathing and other forms of personal care; they can listen and encourage; they can give information and refer" (Twigg 1992, 76).

Although community nurses are potentially key resources to the caregivers, their contribution is limited given the realities of shrinking budgets. There has never been a sufficient number of community nurses to meet the need, and the shortfall will become greater. As caseloads increase, these nurses are likely to cut back on the "social" aspects of caring, focus on the care recipient rather than on both the caregiver and the care recipient, and limit their contact to that which is primarily medical. A second limitation is that these nurses tend to become involved only when there is a health/medical condition. When the care recipient is someone with a mental health problem or is mentally handicapped, the community nurse is not usually involved.

Social workers are the third group of professionals who by training are in a pivotal position to provide supportive services to caregivers. "The training of social workers means that they tend to be more aware of the problems of carers than many other service providers. . . . Social workers are [more likely to be] aware of the potential conflict of interest between the carer and the cared for person" (Twigg 1992, 66). As with community nurses, fewer and fewer social workers are working in community (rather than institutional) agencies and programs. There are exceptions, of course, for example, in the area of child welfare (child abuse treatment and prevention programs) and various programs for persons with severe or chronic mental illness, but fewer agencies are in a position to employ community-based social workers who would provide supportive services to caregivers. Again, in part, this is due to shrinking budgets, managed care, and the difficulty of recovering the costs of the services.

Given these realities, how might we reframe the issue so that professionals are available to caregivers? If professionals are to share responsibility with informal caregivers, it is critical that they understand (a) the capacity and willingness of these caregivers to participate in these transactions, (b) the extent of the support services they provide, and (c) the stress they experience. They must also have an awareness of the needs of the informal caregivers that must be attended to in order that the informal caregivers can fulfill their caregiving functions.

Throughout this book we have argued that not only do many professionals not understand what these caregivers are experiencing, but they have difficulty communicating with them in a meaningful way. This is due in part to the reality that professionals have been socialized to function as the expert—to expect that family members and others involved in the caregiving function will listen to them and take direction from them—and in part to the lack of exposure to the importance of understanding that a caregiver's culture, ethnicity, values, and experiences must be taken into account in the development of relevant supportive services.

The terms *teams* and *team approach* have become common over the past thirty years. They represent a development that initially was concerned with treating the "whole" patient through the organization of multidisciplinary teams. Over time, the team was expanded to include informal caregivers (for example, family members, relatives, and friends) so that they would understand and accept the professionals' treatment plan. Professionals had come to realize that when perceptions of needs differed between them and informal caregivers, the treatment plan tended not to be carried out (Bedard 1967).

Still, involving informal caregivers as members of the team did not necessarily begin with the assumption that all the members were equal partners. In many cases, the informal caregivers were allowed to become a part of the team when the professionals were able to separate out those tasks that required professional expertise and those that did not. The latter tasks were delegated to the "nonprofessional" members of the team, who were allowed to carry them out under the supervision of the professionals. In other instances, the informal caregivers were accepted as fully participating members of the team and were viewed as capable givers of care but also as capable in identifying their own needs rather than relying on professionals to tell them what they needed.

While specialized, technical knowledge and skills will continue to be critical, far more skill in communication, negotiation, and interpersonal sensitivity will be required (McPheeters 1990). Although we did cover this issue at some length in previous chapters, it needs to be raised and highlighted once again. One particularly important element has to do with the highly technical jargon so often used by professionals. Such jargon may be helpful in communicating with professionals in one's own discipline, but it is frequently perceived by care recipients, informal caregivers, and other professionals as a barrier to mutual understanding. In using jargon, the professional creates two barriers ("claims of sincerity and clarity") to achieving meaningful relationships in that the resulting "communication" fails Habermas's test of communicative competency as discussed in chapter 3. It will be important to the development of shared responsibility that professional caregivers communicate in terms that are understandable to others in the caregiving transaction and in ways that are not felt by care recipients or family members as patronizing. The more the professional caregiver has truly assimilated values of respect and mutuality toward others in these transactions, the more likely will these communication efforts succeed, and the less likely they will be perceived as patronizing or intimidating.

All too often, professionals wait until they are asked for information, believing that the responsibility to initiate the dialogue lies with the care recipient or informal caregiver. The professional seems to be operating on the assumption: "If they do not ask questions, they must not have any questions." A variation of this is the professional asking informal caregivers or care recipients whether they have any questions and assuming that if they say no, they actually mean it. These assumptions often have little basis in reality, especially if the professional functions within the Model I framework—that of expert. The professional who operates within a Model II framework, on the other hand, assumes that the informal caregiver and care recipient have a number of questions, and rather than waiting for them to initiate the dialogue, the professional shares with them, in language that is understandable, what he or she is doing, what will be done, and what is likely to happen over the course of service provision. In taking nothing for granted, the professional begins the important process of building a sense of trust in the relationship.

In part, the responsibility to prepare the future practitioner in this more encompassing Model II role lies with educators in the professional schools. Preparation for the process of becoming sensitive to the needs and capabilities of informal caregivers should begin early in the student's training and needs to be addressed in the classroom as well as in the practicum experiences (for example, internships, externships, fieldwork) that most professions require as part of the educational process. This means that the faculty connected to the professional schools must develop real partnerships with the faculty in the practice settings so that the theory of reflective practice can be applied in meaningful ways by the student.

If we are to move in this direction, a number of significant issues need to be addressed. First, the existing curricula in most professional schools tend to focus on the needs of the care receiver—a focus that mirrors the practice in most agencies. Curricula that deal with the needs and strengths of the caregiver are inadequate, in part because the system lacks incentives for the development of such material.

Second, schools have failed to consult informal caregivers about curriculum material, despite the fact that these caregivers can help the professional understand the role that natural networks play. This will probably be the case so long as professionals use academic criteria as the sole criterion for judging the capacity of the informal caregiver to educate the professional.

Finally, we need to develop standards to guide education, since we have yet to define what the provider should know about the informal system with which he or she will interact. As a corollary, professional licensing standards should require this type of training, and professionals should be required to demonstrate their understanding of how this knowledge would shape their practice.

Although much professional training has emphasized team decision making, some training has emphasized the importance of the exercise of independent professional judgment, based on a thorough consideration of technical information about a client (such as medical, psychological, and social histories; assessments of the presenting problem or conditions based on instruments or scales; the development of treatment plans; and in-service settings more similar to those of "solo" practitioners or single categorical programs, such as the practitioner's office or the vocational workshop). The reflective practitioner must be prepared to be more collaborative than autocratic, more willing to negotiate differences rather than dictate orders or actions, and comfortable with the role of partner rather than boss.

A second approach is through continuing professional education for those who have completed school and are now in practice. Through workshops, simulated work environments, or time-limited placement in real-life work settings with clients, their family members, and other providers, experienced practitioners—who previously had not had the opportunity to be exposed to this way of thinking—can broaden their practice orientation.

These learning experiences would need to be carefully structured so as to avoid the misunderstandings and hurt feelings that have frequently plagued interactions between formal and informal caregivers (Biegel, Sales, and Schulz 1991; Goldfarb et al. 1986). Clearly, the earlier that this sort of information can be incorporated into the habits of professional practice, the more likely will it be that professionals and informal caregivers will develop the sort of cooperative partnership advocated in this book. It would seem best if all professional schools would incorporate such information into their curricula and, where appropriate, develop practicum experiences that include informal caregivers.

Empowerment of Caregivers

It once was the norm for consumers passively to accept the instructions, prescriptions, and directives of their formal caregivers without question and, indeed, in many cases, without understanding. This was because consumers and professionals tended to view their relationship as one of the technical expert with authority imparting wisdom to the uninformed or because it was conveyed to the consumer that "that's what the program had to offer." It is now, however, becoming increasingly the norm that the consumer has a much more active voice in the caregiving transaction. This more active voice is manifest in several ways.

Consumer Participation

Consumer participation as a movement is not new. In the human services, consumer participation came into its own in the 1960s, first with the passage of the War on Poverty and then with programs funded by the Model Cities initiative. Under the former program, federal regulations required that the potential recipients of services have representation on decision-making boards. These representatives were seen as valuable sources of information as to what services were needed and how they might be designed so that they were sensitive to the targeted populations. The Model Cities saw this involvement as key to the revitalization of deteriorating neighborhoods.

One of the most significant federal initiatives in the later 1960s was the requirement in the comprehensive health planning legislation that required that 50 percent of local health planning boards be consumers. Over the years, this requirement was tightened to ensure the participation of "real consumers" and not representatives of health care providers.

From these early developments, consumer participation became an essential component on advisory or governing boards of public service agencies at the local, state, and national levels (for example, participation in area agencies on aging, boards of community mental health centers, or members of the Substance Abuse and Mental Health Services Administration National Advisory Council). The initial purpose of this participation in policy development was to help consumers and providers better understand the problems and needs of the target population and the barriers they encountered in obtaining services—whether the services did not exist or, if they did exist, were inaccessible. Efforts to co-locate services, expand hours of operation, simplify application forms, survey consumer opinions, monitor services, and investigate complaints (for instance, through the federally funded, state-operated protection and advocacy offices, which oversee programs for people with developmental disabilities and mental illnesses) are illustrative of changes resulting from consumer participation.

Even though caregivers are "consumers," as a group they have not participated in this movement to the extent that other groups have. If partnerships are to be realized, professionals will need to build outreach services into their ongoing service delivery systems as an integral component. These efforts will help ensure partnerships through the recruitment of caregivers to serve on their agency's boards, administrative teams, and committees in such areas as planning and evaluation.

These partnerships can only be built on a system that recognizes that the satisfaction of the consumer, not the provider of care, is paramount in evaluating the effectiveness of services. The emphasis on consumer satisfaction has been supported by several different changes in the climate of service delivery.

First, the notion of empowerment means that the caregivers' voices must be heard not only in the planning and provision of services but also ultimately in terms of their satisfaction with what has been provided. As a result, caregivers need to insist on the development of ways to express their evaluations.

Second, there has been a corresponding effort for professional caregivers actively to solicit the reactions of caregivers, either through informal inquiry, routine questionnaires during the course of services, or follow-up surveys at the end of defined interventions.

Third, attention to consumer satisfaction has also been stimulated by the broad skepticism that became so prominent in the 1980s regarding the effectiveness of government-run services and by the literature having to do with the reform and "reinvention" of government (for example, Osborne and Gaebler 1992). The growth of interest on the part of local government officials to apply business principles in the public arena, principles that include a major effort to measure outcomes, reintroduces the concern for accountability—being accountable to the public who finance the services and being accountable to the consumers of these services.

Advocacy Efforts

Similar to the consumer participation movement, consumer advocacy has had a fairly long history. Consumer advocacy has aided the effectiveness of the role of consumers at the individual case level and the policy level. There has been rapid growth of organized advocacy for consumer empowerment and the proliferation of organizations and services (such as hot lines, newsletters, pamphlets, books, instructional videos, and self-help clearinghouses) that now empower consumers with knowledge and information about service availability, eligibility requirements, costs, legal rights of consumers, and the like. The *Encyclopedia of Associations* (Daniels and Schwartz 1994) lists hundreds of such organizations and services for virtually any human resource need one can think of.

It is likely that the consumer empowerment movement will continue to permeate all aspects of human service delivery, including further expansion into the private sector. Not only are better informed consumers able to be more equal partners in caregiving transactions, but they are also more likely to insist on such a partnership. They thus encourage practitioners to be more reflective than authoritarian, more Model II than Model I.

A useful distinction may be made between advocacy by consumers per se and advocacy by others on behalf of consumers. The National Mental Health Consumer's self-help clearinghouse is an example of the former, and the National Alliance for the Mentally Ill, consisting of the family members of persons with serious mental illness and professionals, is an example of the latter. The distinction is useful in that the views of these different organizations can sometimes be at odds with one another on some specific issues, while agreeing on other issues. In the examples cited here, both groups agree on issues such as combating stigma and discrimination and urging better coverage of mental illnesses in health insurance plans. They differ on issues such as involuntary commitment and forced medications. Indeed, at times nonprofessional advocates sometimes feel that when professionals advocate for them, they are really advocating for themselves and their agencies and organizations and do not have the best interest of the consumers at heart. In effect, the advocacy can be patronizing—the professionals know what the consumers really need—and can resemble the Model 1 approach.

The strengthening of those organizations currently advocating for caregivers is critical, but since they tend to be specialized in their focus—for example, caregivers providing care to family members with mental illness (NAMI), mental handicap (ARC), Alzheimer's disease, and the frail elderly (the National Alliance for Caregiving)—we need to address the issue of whether these specialized advocacy groups can respond to the new initiatives discussed in chapter 5, or whether it is time to create mechanisms that respond to the generic needs of all caregivers, not as a substitute for the other advocacy groups but as a complementary effort.

Two examples of this more generic type of organization are the National Family Caregivers Association (NFCA) and the National Quality Caregiving Coalition (NQCC) of the Rosalynn Carter Institute. The former is an organization comprising caregivers; the latter is a coalition of organizations concerned with the needs of both formal caregivers and related professionals involved with informal caregivers and care recipients.

Furthermore, given the newly defined role of the states, one that expands their authority to establish priorities and to decide how the block grants will be allocated, traditional advocacy efforts at the national level will have to be channeled to state and local levels. As discussed in the previous chapter, managed care, purchase of service contracting, and performance measurement have serious implications for caregivers.

Unless caregivers become organized and advocate for the programs and services that would support their efforts, they will not be an influential part of the process that makes the important decisions determining what services will be provided under the purchase of service contracts, the amount of services to be covered under purchase of service contracting, and the priority areas for program development that will emerge from the performance measurement initiative. If caregivers are not organized to participate in this political process, not only will their needs not become a priority for future funding, but there are likely to be cutbacks in current resources, as limited as they are.

Recap

The major argument offered in this book is that family members, relatives, friends, and neighbors—the informal caregivers—are providing a great deal of needed care to people who are unable to meet all of their own needs. The evidence to support this conclusion is overwhelming. Furthermore, since they are providing this care, demands on the formal system are less than it might be otherwise. They are providing this care, however, at great personal cost.

We have also been concerned about the nature of caregiving and introduced the distinction between caregiving and caring, suggesting that in some instances, caregiving can be limited to meeting the instrumental needs of the care recipient. Caregiving may not be "caring" in the sense that Mayeroff, Parker, Graham, and Leira have discussed the concept.

We identified some of the reasons that the caregiver may not be caring and suggested that the formal system can play a major role in supporting the caregiver so that the relationship between the giver and the recipient might go beyond minimal provision of concrete care. In fact, we would argue that unless the formal system develops responsive supportive services, those who now "care" will inevitably redefine their role to include only the provision of instrumental services, and in time many will transfer the caregiving function to the formal system.

Finally, we pointed out that the issue goes far beyond the problem of scarce resources so often used as an excuse for not developing supportive services for caregivers. While additional resources are necessary, they will be largely ineffective if professionals do not change their approach to informal caregivers. Ideally, partnerships can be formed at both the service delivery level as well as the policy level. To do so, professionals need to expand their practice base. They need to take on the role of the reflective practitioner—to participate in the empowering process, to assist caregivers in becoming more independent rather than remaining in a dependency relationship with the professional. The key is to foster a sense of shared responsibility, interdependency, trust, and mutual respect—to help bring about the Caring Society.

> The basic value assertion or first principle of the Caring Society is that human social development—defined as the continual broadening of human experience and perfection of human social relations over the life cycle—should be the aim of society. We should strive in the present to develop ourselves and our children into socially competent people, into better and better future citizens, into citizens who will create and support a just, democratic, human, and caring community and social order. Thus, we speak of the Competent Society as well as the Caring Society. (Moroney and Dokecki 1984, 229)

Appendix A

Definitions of Caregivers

Formal (professional) caregivers provide health care and/or social services to others as a function of their chosen profession using skills, knowledge, and insights obtained primarily through formal training. The amount of education required to be certified in various professions varies greatly. Individuals serving in administrative or academic positions who have been trained in the helping professions are also considered caregivers because their orientation and actions significantly impact front-line care providers. Usually, formal caregivers receive financial compensation for their services, but sometimes they do not in a situation where they serve as volunteers to organizations, groups, or individuals. Caregivers in the formal system directly address health care needs by providing concrete services, knowledge, and advice; however, they may also provide social support or counseling.

Informal (lay or family) caregivers provide care and assistance to others without financial or material gain. Usually, this service occurs in the context of an ongoing relationship and is an expression of concern and love for a relative, friend, or fellow human being. Caregivers in the informal system help partially or completely dependent people on a regular basis with activities of daily living such as dressing, feeding, managing finances, transportation, administering medicines, or meal preparation. They also frequently provide love, affection, intimacy, and social support.

Volunteer caregivers may be considered as formal (professional) or informal (lay or family) depending on the formal training received and specific job as a volunteer. An example of a formal volunteer caregiver is a nurse who works for a hospice (as a nurse) with no pay. An informal volunteer caregiver might be a church volunteer who visits elderly persons and "shut-ins" as part of an ongoing church-supported program.

Dual caregivers are formal caregivers who also care for family members or relatives, outside their professional responsibility.

Appendix B

Characteristics, Concerns, and Concrete Needs of Formal and Informal Caregivers: The CARE-NET Study

When an organization is required to justify its existence or makes a request for funding, a needs assessment of the client/consumer population is undertaken. So too when an organization wishes to ensure that it is on target in serving its clients, a needs assessment is in order. In this regard the West Central Georgia Caregivers' Network (CARE-NET) Leadership Council was no different from other organized groups. Very early in its existence, the council determined that a needs assessment was essential in setting priorities for programs and assistance for caregivers in the region served by the network. CARE-NET departed from the usual approaches to conducting needs assessments, however, in seeking serious involvement of caregivers, CARE-NET leaders, regional educational institutions, and Rosalynn Carter Institute (RCI) staff members. The project became more than simply a needs assessment; it became a study of the issues, concerns, problems, and needs of caregivers.

The CARE-NET study was unique in at least six ways. First, there was a concentration on the characteristics, problems, and needs of formal caregivers in general. Numerous efforts have been directed toward understanding discrete groups of formal caregivers such as psychologists, psychiatrists, nurses, and social workers, but the similarities among these caregivers in the formal system have seldom been explored as they were in the CARE-NET project. Second, an attempt was made to determine and understand the needs of lay caregivers—people in the informal system who provide assistance to individuals with emotional and mental problems, physical illnesses, difficulties associated with aging, and developmental disabilities. Third, the study compared the generic caregiving needs found in the formal and informal systems. Fourth, whereas many studies have considered the personal outcomes of the caregiving process (stress reactions, depression, hostility, perceived burden, burnout), we placed greater emphasis on the caregiving process itself and the array of needs that caregivers experience. Fifth, we employed both quantitative surveys and qualitative interviews. Finally, we involved consumers and front-line health care providers in the process of planning the study and used approaches that ensured that stakeholders in the informal and formal caregiving systems communicated and developed better connections with each other. The interview itself provided the means for an important three-way exchange of information between formal caregivers, informal caregivers, and students (future caregivers), thereby creating the opportunity for increased understanding and appreciation among all three points of view.

The research project was designed and conducted to represent contextualist epistemology, an approach that, in the words of James Kelly (1990), "encourages the researcher and participant to collaborate in conjoint understanding of the phenomena of shared interest. Phenomena are considered to be defined according to the experience of the participants, including their relationship with the researcher" (772). It is this emphasis on process as well as outcomes that most distinguishes the CARE-NET research project from previous efforts. The interview process and degree of involvement of caregivers in planning are models for the collaborative approach of the RCI, under whose auspices the CARE-NET Leadership Council operates in pursuing its mission.

Important to the planning process was the recognition that (1) formal and informal caregivers are involved in essentially identical goals and tasks and (2) many barriers impede communication between the two groups in the everyday world. Opening channels of communication between the formal and informal systems of caregiving became a major objective of the project. Thus, the process of data gathering itself was planned as one means of fulfilling that objective. In the first phase of the study, informal caregivers were teamed with students to interview formal caregivers. In the second phase, students and formal caregivers conducted interviews with informal caregivers. This approach facilitated communication between formal and informal caregivers and acquainted potential caregivers, the students, with various aspects of caregiving.

Details about the development of the interview questions and items for the written questionnaires are available from the RCI. What is especially significant about the process is the integral involvement at all stages of its development by area caregivers and institute staff, who designed the interviews and questionnaires to address five primary areas: burnout in caregiving; preparatory and continuing education for the caregiving role; relationships between all the persons involved in a caregiving situation; status and recognition/general morale of caregivers; and concrete needs (financial, transportation, legal, and so on). Ultimately, 98 formal caregivers—defined as the persons who provide or direct the provision of health care and/or social services as a function of their chosen profession using skills, knowledge, and insights obtained primarily through formal training—were interviewed about their caregiving situations, concerns, and needs. They and 158 others also completed written questionnaires. These 256 participants were selected through a random sampling process from 2,650 formal caregivers in the sixteen-county region. The professional specialties represented were quite diverse, as indicated by the job titles given, some of which were service coordinator, licensed practical nurse, program director, physician, psychologist, director of family and children services, social services specialist, counselor, house parent, marriage and family therapist, caseworker, human service technician, administrator, chaplain, social worker, certified nursing assistant, medical assistant, nurse's aide, and instructor. Five hundred forty-three informal caregivers from the same region were identified, and a random sample of 49 were interviewed about their caregiving situations, concerns, and needs. A total of 175 informal caregivers, including those who were interviewed, completed written questionnaires.

Because of the number of caregivers involved and the participatory process by which the research was designed and carried out, the CARE-NET study gleaned invaluable information about the nature of caregiving and about caregivers' needs and concerns. We cannot be certain, of course, that our participants were fully representative of caregivers in CARE-NET's sixteen-county region or across the nation, that the right questions were asked in ways that would allow honest and candid responses, or how closely the research methodology was always followed by those involved in the study's design and data collection. These and similar issues should provide direction for future research. Nevertheless, the CARE-NET study produced an excellent picture of caregivers who are actively engaged in caring for ill or disabled individuals.

Characteristics of Caregivers

Formal Caregivers

Seventy-two percent of the formal caregivers randomly selected to participate in the CARE-NET study were women, and 28 percent were men. Women delivered most of the direct care and service to patients and clients, with many of the men filling supervisory and administrative posts; 59 percent of the men and 38 percent of the women held management-level positions. Sixty-three percent of this group of participants were white and 37 percent black. The length of time they had worked as formal caregivers varied greatly, with 23 percent having less than five years of experience and 22 percent having more than twenty years of experience. The majority of the formal caregivers indicated that they spent a great deal of time involved in direct or primary care to patients or clients.

Formal caregivers representing all professional backgrounds offered impressive accounts of their caregiving experiences. Common positive experiences included saving lives, helping people remain in the community, finding suitable housing for clients, connecting clients with needed community resources, and receiving the gratitude of persons they had helped. A nurse said that interacting with the patients was the most desirable feature of her work: "I like the emotional and spiritual aspects of caregiving better than the medical." A nursing assistant in a skilled nursing facility described her work experience similarly: "I enjoy my job very much and get along well with my co-workers. However, patient care is the most important, which includes showing your love and giving respect."

Formal caregivers also gave accounts of unmet expectations, abuse of children and older adults, deaths of patients, sudden turns for the worse, lack of family involvement in treatment, too few resources, and frustrations with bureaucratic barriers to effective caregiving. It seems that despite their length of service, all formal caregivers have experienced disappointments and failures during their careers, but for most, the wealth of enriching experiences apparently outweighs the disappointments.

A variety of life experiences seems to lead formal caregivers to their career choices. According to information obtained in the CARE-NET interviews, they can be grouped in four categories:

1. *History of family caregiving or dysfunction.* Approximately two-thirds of the formal caregivers interviewed identified a personal history of informal caregiving. These experiences in caregiving ranged from time-limited episodes of assisting an ill loved one to serving as primary caregiver for one or more disabled family members. Other formal caregivers described informal caregiving experiences but related examples that might be defined as providing moral support to a friend or loved one, such as talking to a family member going through a divorce. Many described experiences providing personal care to relatives prior to becoming formal caregivers. One individual, for example, commented that her family had always relied on her to play the supportive, helping role. Whether one had provided hands-on caregiving or one's helping role had been less well structured, the role of caregiver was defined as familial for many individuals. In a related vein, several formal caregivers discussed histories of family problems that led them to want to help others in similar situations, and 31 percent had family members currently requiring care.

2. *Personal problems.* Several formal caregivers said that their own previous needs for care had led them into helping professions. A few individuals cited a history of psychotherapy that was instrumental in their decision to enter caregiving.

3. *Personal values.* A number of formal caregivers indicated that they had chosen to enter a helping profession because of the values represented in caregiving. Some spoke of it as a calling, one as "a destiny." One said that her caregiving career grew out of missionary experiences, and others commented on the desirability of helping others. A unique perspective was offered by one caregiver, who stated, "I think there's a genetic factor involved. You're born a caring person."

4. *Serendipity.* Many formal caregivers indicated that they had not consciously chosen a caregiving field but had accepted jobs that were offered and remained in the field because they enjoyed it. One person described his vocation as something he "sort of fell into."

As indicated above, a history of family caregiving often contributes to the choice of caregiving as a professional career, and it often influences the manner in which a formal caregiver approaches her or his work. When asked about the ways in which their informal caregiving experiences affected their professional provision of care, individuals responded in various ways, with most answers relating to the impact of this historical factor on their perspectives and attitudes. Only a small minority felt that their personal caregiving experiences had not directly affected their formal attitudes or behavior, and no one indicated a negative influence of informal caregiving. Most stated that experiences heightened their empathy and understanding in their professional duties. One remarked, "When people say, 'We're through' or 'I can't deal with this anymore,' I can understand." And another: "It's made me more aware and more sensitive to the needs of my patients and their feelings."

Informal Caregivers

As defined earlier, informal caregivers may be providing care for an immediate family member, another relative, a neighbor, or a friend. Most frequently named as recipients of care among the CARE-NET study's participants were mothers, sons, and husbands. Six percent of the caregivers indicated that they were providing care for a friend. Eighty percent of the informal caregivers were women. Seventy-one percent of the group were white and 29 percent black. Black informal caregivers were underrepresented in the study, as black persons make up 41 percent of the population in CARE-NET's geographic area.

When caregivers were asked to indicate the nature of the problem requiring their care, the three most often mentioned were developmental disability, physical illness, and problems related to aging. Mental illness and substance abuse were also represented. Some care recipients, of course, were affected by two or more problems. Fifty-six percent of the caregivers reported that they were assisting someone aged sixty-one or older, but all age groups were represented, as shown in table B.1.

TABLE B.1. Age of Person Being Cared For

Age	Percentage of Caregivers
0–18 years	12%
19–30 years	10%
31–45 years	13%
46–60 years	9%
61 years and over	56%

The amount of time spent in caregiving activities each week ranged from two or three hours to well over forty hours. Forty-one percent of informal caregivers indicated that they spent more than forty hours each week—the equivalent of a full-time job—providing care. Many of these saw their caregiving as an around-the-clock responsibility.

The effects of intense responsibility in caregiving are increased by the duration of the caregiving experience, according to the CARE-NET study participants. The largest percentage of caregivers—35 percent—reported more than ten years in their current caregiving situation. An elderly woman who cares for her physically ill husband stated it aptly: "I have been on 24-hour duty for 22 years."

The kinds of caregiving assistance provided by informal caregivers are quite varied. Our participants reported being involved in the following types of care: emotional support (71 percent of the caregivers), transportation (67 percent), housekeeping (65 percent), providing meals (65 percent), sit with/accompany (62 percent), physical health care (53 percent), personal hygiene (48 percent), lifting/assisting with movement (39 percent), advocacy (27 percent), and other activities (17 percent). It is notable that many of these tasks are taxing and sometimes unpleasant. Many may also be rewarding, to the extent that burnout is not a factor. Let us look at three brief accounts of caregivers' activities and perspectives:

I spend all day caring for my son. I feel so obligated. Daily activities include getting him out of bed, transporting for guitar lessons, having to be at home for him all the time, making sure he takes his medications, and struggling to teach him a value system.

I spend all day and sometimes half of the night taking care of my brother. I give him his meals, watch him, wash his clothes and bathe him. I exercise his leg to keep the circulation going, so he won't have to have it amputated. I give him his medication, take him to the doctor once a month, and to Adult Mental Health Clinic every six months. I provide all the transportation.

Due to the crippling effects of the disease, my husband required absolutely total care. He didn't want anyone but me, and I thought I was supposed to do it all. At the time, I was self-employed. I moved my business and my entire life to take care of him and renovated the house to meet his needs. Total care means bathing, dressing, feeding, lifting, etc.

Even though the three above accounts vary in terms of the caregiving relationships and difficulties of the care receiver, all describe the sometimes demanding nature of caregiving and the variety of tasks required of the caregiver. Indeed, they illustrate just how much of the informal caregiver's life may be devoted to caregiving activities. A large number (45 percent) of the study's lay participants reported that they had assumed total responsibility for caregiving, and 28 percent reported responsibility for "most" of the recipient's care. Most of the care was provided by these caregivers in their own homes or in the home of the care recipient. The informal caregivers who were interviewed saw themselves as busy people, often juggling multiple roles and responsibilities. "Hectic" is a word used frequently by caregivers to describe their schedules. Several reported handling caregiving responsibilities for both immediate and extended family members. The group often reported having little spare time, with most of their activities centering around the demands of caregiving, and frequently feeling too tired to enjoy rest and relaxation when time becomes available. Many, in fact, reported that they volunteered time for outside caregiving activities. Only a minority of the caregivers reported a wide variety of interests in which they engaged, and these generally responded more positively to their caregiving roles. It appears, then, that the ability of caregivers to care for themselves bears a closer relationship to the degree of their satisfaction as caregivers than does the amount of time spent in caregiving, the number of individuals cared for, the amount of disruption to the home, or other quantitative factors.

The degree to which caregivers function well in their demanding roles may be at least partially, if not greatly, dependent on the supports available to them. Such supports may be familial, organizational, professional, casual, or spiritual. Some informal caregivers are clearly able to identify supports available to them, whereas others either have no one else available or perceive others as being unresponsive to their needs. Most look to immediate family members for assistance, but the family is not always able to provide the support that is needed or requested. Informal caregivers in this study reported receiving the greatest amount of assistance from their spouses (24 percent), their daughters (18 percent), and their sons (16 percent).

Results of the CARE-NET study indicated, however, that some caregivers called on assistance from others only reluctantly or had criticism of how others managed the caregiving duties that they normally performed themselves. Others criticized the amount of caregiving that others were willing to provide. They reported that relatives living close to the care recipient were most likely to assist with caregiving responsibilities and that logistical considerations tended to limit the extent to which other family members were routinely engaged in the caregiving process.

Considerations of privacy also limit the range of resources used by many informal caregivers. Only 9 percent of our sample said that they most often turned to public agencies for assistance, and 9 percent said that they usually sought help from private agencies; in terms of actual assistance received, only 49 percent of the informal caregivers reported receiving some sort of caregiving assistance from formal caregivers or agency programs. Most prefer to seek assistance from other family members, neighbors, or church associates, for reasons that are summarized in one individual's comment: "I don't turn to outside people because they want to know your business but not share your problems." Relying on other laypersons for additional support or respite has its pitfalls, however. The availability of family and friends can change unexpectedly, and continually asking for help of the same group of people requires a great deal of assertiveness on the part of the primary caregiver. When asked for the advice they would give to other informal caregivers, many members of the CARE-NET sample noted the necessity of seeking assistance from others, despite the difficulties inherent in such reliances. "People shouldn't be martyrs," one asserted. "Take time for yourself. Ask for help in the home," advised another. A third said, "Don't think you are the only one who can provide care; share the responsibility of care; demand help from family members."

For noncustodial help and moral support, informal caregivers identified a wide variety of resources, including friends, agencies, formal support groups, and God. Religious and family associates were the most frequently mentioned sources of support, and almost half of the informal caregivers who were interviewed identified important sources of spiritual support, including their church community. Formal agency supports were mentioned far less frequently. Similarly, organized support and advocacy groups were mentioned, but many caregivers indicated that they have found comparable avenues of support through more informal means. One representative caregiver described her extended support system in terms of informally based associations: "I have a couple of friends, both of my sisters, and my daughter who support me. I feel well supported. I have four cats who are a big help. I love my work. It's very restorative. I also have my minister. . . . I have lots of interaction with others."

The question of caregiving alternatives—what would happen if the current caregiver could no longer provide care—was a vexing one to many informal caregivers. The most frequent option identified was other family members or relatives followed by a nursing home or other institutional care. Also cited were church, trust arrangements, boarding homes, and paid attendants. Only three of the forty-nine informal caregivers who were interviewed mentioned state or government assistance.

Many informal caregivers expressed a high degree of anxiety about such potential changes in care, both for themselves and for the care recipient. Their responses included the following statements: "I would be lost." "It would be a very traumatic experience." "I would worry myself to death." "It's difficult to talk about." "It would destroy [the care recipient]." "It would be a difficult burden." "It would devastate me and my family." "I don't want to think about it." A few caregivers expressed concerns about the survival of their loved one, and there was a pervasive theme that no one could or would do the job as well or as willingly as they had. One caregiver expounded, "I would be very unhappy and worried for a long time about whether others were doing as good a job. . . . My family would fall apart. I do not believe my daughter has the ability to give like I do. It would destroy my family. It would destroy my daughter's marriage. It would destroy my daughter. I have always assumed I would be there for him. Everyone feels he is my responsibility."

In many cases, the reality is that there is no adequate alternative to the caregiving provided by the current primary caregiver. Citing financial considerations, lack of family availability or willingness to assist, and other factors, many family caregivers find themselves without reasonable alternatives. Some voice despair at this plight, but much pride about what they personally have been able to accomplish is also commonly heard. A small number of caregivers, in contrast, anticipate some feelings of relief at being able to relinquish the caregiving role.

Two areas of a caregiver's life that are often vulnerable to the negative impact of caregiving are financial and employment situations. Family caregivers often spoke of the expense involved in caregiving in terms of sacrifices made by the rest of the family. "Our lives have changed from comfortable to a life of survival," said one. Another commented that "often times there was not enough to go around to other family members. There are things that I would like to do . . . but can't." Others described their caregiving as causing "severe financial stress" or as having interfered with "financial plans." Half the informal caregivers in the CARE-NET study reported that they or their care recipients received financial assistance, primarily from government programs, that was directly helpful in their caregiving situation. A few said that they were helped financially by family members or by the care recipient. About half described the assistance they received as adequate.

More than a quarter of the informal caregivers reported that their caregiving duties had caused problems for them at work. Many stated that their caregiving activities had caused them to miss work; over one-third reported an absence of more than one month. It is encouraging to note that 50 percent of the caregivers reported no repercussions from their absence, and 33 percent were permitted to use their sick leave. Some, however, were fired or lost income as a result of their absences. For most caregivers, employers had shown a degree of support or tolerance, and the impact on their employment or careers was subtle. Others commented that caregiving responsibilities had caused career opportunities to be curtailed.

Burden and Reward, Love and Duty

A nagging question in the study of caregivers from the formal and informal arenas has been the relative extent to which the activities and responsibilities of assisting another person are perceived as being rewarding or burdensome. An overwhelmingly large proportion of our formal and informal caregivers reported caregiving to be rewarding. However, many more informal caregivers (21 percent) than formal ones (6 percent) also saw caregiving activities as a burden. In a sense, then, and particularly for informal caregivers, the process of caregiving is not unlike running a marathon that one finds arduous but also satisfying.

Perhaps a large degree of the reward of caregiving comes from a sense that a duty has been carried out or that a mission inspired by love for another person has been accomplished. Narrative descriptions given by two caregivers help to illustrate this sense of duty fulfilled. One caregiver wrote, "I love my mother dearly. I would take care of her no matter how stressed or depressed I became. I am not a certified caretaker. It's just a natural response to help because of the love and sense of duty I feel to a family member." The other wrote of her situation, "As the eldest of five living children, I took responsibility because the others wouldn't, a decision which cost my health, my job and more than likely, my marriage. I care for her out of love and duty."

The fact that more informal than formal caregivers find the task burdensome is likely attributable to the fact that family members act as caregivers twenty-four hours a day and cannot resign from the task. It is significant to note in this regard that according to our study, family members who are caregivers generally believe that they should take primary responsibility for the burden of caregiving. Only 20 percent of these caregivers said they sought any help with their burden, and 24 percent reported that their caregiving made them feel depressed or sad. Some caregivers were quite vocal about the harsh realities of caregiving and their own frustrations with it.

A sizable majority of our formal caregivers indicated that their caregiving experiences had been rewarding. Many saw themselves doing a job that had to be done and growing from the experience in the process. Several noted that their fulfillment came from the actual experience of giving care, and one commented on the fulfillment in receiving emotional feedback from patients. The intrinsic rewards are tempered for many of these caregivers, however, by frustrations with required paperwork, financial concerns, and regulatory problems. The extent to which a caregiver finds caregiving to be rewarding or burdensome may be related to the perceived voluntary or involuntary nature of the responsibility, especially for informal caregivers. For formal caregivers there is almost always a considerable degree of choice about the pursuit of a caregiving profession. For informal caregivers, the issue of choice is more complex and often relates to the sense of duty that they feel. Some informal caregivers defined their caregiving as voluntary because it was the only alternative to institutionalization for their loved ones—an alternative they had chosen. Others considered the same situation to have forced them by default into caregiving roles. Many indicated ambivalence about their "forced choice." One stated, "It's entirely voluntary. I do not deal with guilt well." Others made similar responses, such as, "Voluntary—but no other choice." Reasons for accepting the role of caregiver included family loyalty, moral obligation, and lack of other resources. A few caregivers indicated that they had actively volunteered for their responsibilities, even though alternatives were available. Overall, it was found that satisfaction with the informal caregiving role is clearly related to one's perception of the degree of choice involved in it.

Most people would agree that caregiving makes a great difference in the lives of those receiving care. It is clear here that helping others also makes a great difference in the lives of the caregivers as well. Almost all formal caregivers, for example, stated that their ideas about caregiving had changed during their careers. For some, but not all, these changes brought greater satisfaction. Many described increases in their understanding, compassion, empathy, knowledge, skill, and wisdom. "I've learned that it's really not just a job . . . but a commitment," said one caregiver, who stated further, "I'm now more motivated and I care more about the concerns of others than when I first stated my career." A physician expressed it in this way: "My caregiving has changed due to the fact that I now have a better understanding of the human side of caregiving rather than the medical side."

Another theme in the formal caregivers' responses was their loss of idealism and development of a more realistic, objective, or detached perspective. One explained, "I have become hardened to problems. I have worked up a defense mechanism because you can only give so much without being totally empty." Another said, "You can't be idealistic and survive. You have to accept a lot less than you prefer in every aspect."

Informal caregivers expressed a variety of feelings as they described the difference caregiving had made in their lives. For some, the difference was unwelcome and stressful—for example, "It has enhanced Mother's life and brought mine down." Some acknowledged feelings of resentment, frustration, and tragedy that had developed after long-term caregiving.

Family role reversals and other changes in familial relationships were particularly difficult for some of the caregivers, as was their initial surprise about the breadth and depth of the responsibilities they had incurred. "It's changed our relationship," commented one woman about caring for her disabled husband. "I'm no longer the wife, I'm the mother. My husband acts like a child, constantly asking me for things . . . and he depends on me to make all decisions." Other caregivers, however, spoke of important life lessons they had learned, such as accepting others' uniqueness, changing their personal priorities, gaining increased respect for life. Some noted an increase in their empathy, compassion, patience, frustration tolerance, and respect for caregivers and for those needing care. One person summed up the change by stating her understanding that caregiving "is more important than many other things in life."

Education and training were seen by many caregivers, especially informal ones, as a form of support that is needed but in short supply. More than half of the informal caregivers and a third of those in the formal system reported inadequate opportunities to attend workshops, seminars, and conferences related to caregiving. Informal caregivers most often identified their educational needs as falling into the following categories: broader knowledge of specific illnesses or disabilities; coping skills/emotional support; health, medical, or medication information; accessing services/availability of services; "how-tos" of caregiving; and legal or regulatory information. The types of training and educational needs identified by formal caregivers were quite varied but generally comprised these categories: training in the specific disabilities or illnesses; treatment issues; management/leadership training; current research and technology; and professional development.

Most formal and informal caregivers expressed an interest in continuing their education and training in caregiving. The primary similarity in their learning interests was their concern about obtaining more in-depth information about specific illnesses or disabilities. Otherwise, informal caregivers were more interested in generic skills and information, while formal caregivers expressed greater interest in technical, issue-oriented, and other professional areas. They noted the importance of being involved in a continuous learning process and stated in resounding numbers that "academic institutions could do more to help caregivers."

More effective communication among the caregivers involved with an individual recipient of care was also noted to be an important need. Although both formal and informal caregivers indicated that they trusted fellow caregivers, that they received adequate support from their own families, and that they were able to connect with fellow caregivers in meaningful ways, fewer than 60 percent agreed that there was effective communication among all parties involved in the caregiving process. When asked to describe good and bad experiences with formal caregivers, the dominant issue raised by informal caregivers was communication and information sharing. One-third of them described concern with formal caregivers' communication, including the extent to which they listen or appear to listen to both the informal caregiver and the care recipient. They valued greatly the formal caregiver who listens to others' needs and provides relevant information. Formal caregivers likewise emphasized the need for more and better communication between informal and formal caregivers. Yet there was significant disparity between the two groups' responses to questions about representatives of the formal system sharing pertinent information with informal caregivers. The suggestion is that, by and large, formal caregivers do offer relevant information about technical matters and support services, but not in a manner that can be digested by or is useful to informal caregivers. However, both groups heavily endorsed the need for greater cooperation between agencies and formal caregivers in order to provide people with better services.

Less than two-thirds of the study participants stated a belief that members of the other group (family members for formal caregivers; professionals and agency representatives for the informal caregivers) were able and willing to assist in the care of patients or clients. This may be related to the lack of adequate communication and collaboration between formal and informal systems. A man who cares for his sister made this disturbing comment: "I feel government agencies don't give a damn. I've been given the bum's rush many times; resources seem to always lead to dead ends. I keep up a front for my sister's sake, but depression never goes away. The system is a sad, sick joke."

When formal caregivers were asked about their views on the roles and responsibilities of family members, they usually demonstrated a great deal of respect for the informal caregiving role. Many, however, expressed concerns about family members' reluctance to be involved in provision of care at all stages of the process, while others felt that families should distance themselves from the caregiving process and allow their care recipient greater independence and responsibility. Similarly, attitudes of informal caregivers toward formal caregivers were rarely neutral. Many shared "horror stories" about agencies, institutions, or individual formal caregivers; others identified specific formal caregivers who had made their loved ones' lives easier.

When asked what they saw as the major needs of informal caregivers, formal caregivers offered a wide variety of suggestions ranging from concrete needs to qualities of character. The major need identified was for training, education, or information, followed by a need for support groups or other support systems and a need for respite care. Many formal caregivers offered philosophical advice to all caregivers about the need to maintain emotional equilibrium. Specific suggestions for family members were for patience and understanding, commitment to the patient, the need to push the patient back to health, the need to understand that one does not need to feel guilty, the need to set and enforce personal limits, awareness of the road to burnout, and learning to take care of oneself.

Informal caregivers' advice to formal caregivers primarily involved attitudinal or stylistic concerns, rather than the actual care provided. They frequently cited the need for greater sensitivity, empathy, and compassion among formal caregivers. "Love comes to mind," one woman responded when asked what formal caregivers need in order to do their professional jobs better. General advice offered to formal caregivers by informal caregivers included the following:

- ∾ Doctors need to be told that the emotional and physical are both important.

- ∾ TLC will go further than all the medication you can give.

- ∾ Respect the informal caregiver.

- ∾ Treat others as you would be treated.

- ∾ I don't want to be patronized.

Indeed, 51 percent of the formal caregivers surveyed indicated that they did not have sufficient time to consult with families regarding how they might assist with the care of their patients or clients. The important question here is "why?" Are there too many other demands on formal caregivers? Do our contemporary, bureaucratic settings for provision of care interfere with helping? In this regard, 61 percent of the formal caregivers agreed that the bureaucratic orientation and excessive paperwork required in their organizations kept them from being effective on the job. Their most frequently mentioned complaint was "too much paperwork." A more disturbing possibility is that some formal caregivers do not value the potential contributions of family caregivers and therefore do not "make time" to connect with them. Our interviews with formal caregivers showed that some do believe families should, in essence, let the formal caregivers do their job—that too much family involvement "muddies the works."

Nevertheless, both formal and informal caregivers reported that they feel respected and admired and that they had received recommendations from other persons because of their caregiving roles. Twenty-nine percent of the informal caregivers and 43 percent of the formal caregivers said that they had received recognition in the news media. About 60 percent of the formal caregivers' agencies were said to have received media recognition. Seeking emotional support, on the other hand, carries a stigma for both groups of caregivers. More than one-third of formal caregivers and 27 percent of informal caregivers believed that they would be viewed negatively if they sought counseling. These responses appear to demonstrate a need for greater advocacy for caregivers and a increased public understanding of the multifaceted rigors of the caregiving experience.

One of the major pitfalls of caregiving is the high probability of burnout. Half of the informal caregivers and more than a third of the formal caregivers reported that they were "probably experiencing burnout." Even greater numbers of both groups indicated that they "feel used up at the end of the day" and often "feel just plain exhausted." They commented on "work overload," "not [having] enough time," having to "work too hard," being fatigued, and working with not enough staff. One formal caregiver commented, "The work is demanding; people don't realize how much it takes of their personal life. It takes a lot of energy to give so intensely to people." More indications of burnout were demonstrated among younger workers than among older ones. We can only speculate that older formal caregiver have come to grips with the process of burnout and learned ways to avoid the downward spiral. An informal caregiver similarly noted, "The pressure I'm under—taking care of everything myself—the car, the house, the finances; it's constant pressure." Many informal caregivers also acknowledged that they had few outlets for coping with stress. Three variables were found to be associated with informal caregivers' level of burnout: assistance received by the caregiver, the caregivers' responsibility for personal hygiene of the care recipient, and importance of formal religious beliefs to the caregiver; but our analyses do not point to a single major variable that accounts for burnout. It appears that caregivers who receive assistance tend to have lower burnout rates than those without assistance, that caregivers who assist with personal hygiene (bathing, dressing, and bodily functions) tend to have higher rates of burnout, and that those for whom religion is very important have a considerably lower rate of burnout. Caregivers often mentioned their religious faith as both a source of strength and a source of meaningful, relaxing activities that help them to rest and revitalize from rigors of caregiving.

These results point out the importance to caregivers of support and assistance with their duties. Respite care alternatives would provide physical and mental relief, and help in attending to the personal hygiene of the person receiving care may be most useful and appreciated. The role of the church in helping caregivers to cope appears to be important already and may provide a basis for enhancement of support and respite services. Seventy percent of informal caregivers stated that their churches' spiritual guidance helped with their caregiving, and 86 percent described their religious beliefs as very important.

Family caregivers frequently expressed reliance on spiritual supports, citing prayer and belief in God as major sources of strength. Nearly as many formal caregivers also noted that religious beliefs hold important positions in their lives. Perhaps this dispels a commonly held notion that formal caregivers are mostly atheists, agnostics, or secular humanists. On the other hand, many of the persons surveyed live in what is often described as the "Bible Belt," so these results may not be representative.

When asked, however, about concrete assistance received from their churches—such as transportation, money, or supplies—only 10 percent of the informal caregivers indicated that the church provided such resources, and many felt that their churches did not provide adequate help to caregivers, although a number of individual exceptions were noted; that is, there were many individual examples of concrete assistance provided by church volunteers. Further documentation of tangible help provided by churches in such areas as health care, counseling, housing,

TABLE B.2. Comparative Rankings of Needs by Formal and Informal Caregivers

Formal Caregivers Resource/Activity		Informal Caregivers Resource/Activity	
1	Peer-support groups available to professional caregivers	1	Community resources
2	Personal counseling available to professional caregivers	2	Linkage with other caregivers
3	Availability of sufficient staff to caregivers	3	Personal counseling available
4	Salary received	4	Availability of people to assist with caregiving
5	Community resources	5	Linkage with professional caregivers
6	Linkage with family caregivers	6	Specialized training
7	Specialized training	7	Financial assistance
8	Stability in work environment	8	Time away from caregiving responsibilities
9	Respect provided by others	9	Availability of people in similar situations to support each other
10	More referral resources (programs or people)	10	Information

and programs for elderly persons has been presented in a recent study by Miller (1993).

Concrete needs of both formal and informal caregivers were rank-ordered by the researchers based on the caregivers' ratings as to their current availability and future importance. The lists of most-needed resources for the two groups bear striking similarities, particularly in the importance placed on interpersonal linkages and support, personal counseling, and persons available to assist with caregiving.

Formal and informal caregivers seem to place great value on linkage with each other. A closer look at our data reveals that caregivers do not perceive an inadequacy of linkage activities currently, but they place importance on greater linkages for meeting future needs. This provides an indication of hope for the likelihood of increased convergence of the two caregiving groups in the future to form effective caregiving partnerships.

What We Have Learned

Results of the CARE-NET study demonstrate clearly that caregivers are tenacious but vulnerable. Both formal and informal caregivers carry out their jobs day by day, often with inadequate interaction with each other, with insufficient assistance, and in the face of stress that can lead to burnout. It is our hope that this study will have an impact that extends far beyond the bounds of west central Georgia, where the caregivers' network is beginning to address the needs of caregivers with new programs and through the heightened understanding and appreciation that formal and informal caregivers there have developed for each other. The collaborative process through which the study was conducted has resulted in more open communication, empathy, and new alliances among formal caregivers, informal caregivers, and the academic community, and the knowledge that it allowed us to obtain has brought about the following changes in our community:

1. Heightened awareness on the part of formal caregivers of the concerns, problems, and issues facing informal caregivers.

2. Increased public awareness of who is a caregiver and the concept of the generic caregiving.

3. Increased public awareness of the rewards and burdens of caregiving.

4. Greater understanding and acceptance of the emotional support needed by both formal and informal caregivers in order to prevent or minimize the effects of burnout.

5. Increased attention to issues related to gender, cultural diversity, and age and their influence on caregiving roles and responsibilities.

6. Increased acceptance by formal caregivers of informal caregivers as valuable members of the "caregiving team."

7. Encouragement of the academic and research organizations to conduct further study of the issues, problems, and concerns faced by caregivers.

Perhaps the potential impact of the CARE-NET study can be illustrated best by its impact on some of the project's interviewers. One commented, "I will carry it with me the rest of my life." Another interviewer, a student, had this insightful response: "I realize that I'll probably have to take care of my parents some day. I will be more careful how I handle it and consider their feelings more when the time comes." And a formal caregiver who had interviewed a family caregiver said simply, "She touched my heart." Such evidence of people's ability to glean mutual understanding and respect on the basis of a single project says much about our potential to enhance caregiving by providing appropriate instrumental and emotional support to those who provide care.

Notes

1. Our approach to defining and elaborating the nature of caring is guided mainly by Milton Mayeroff's classic on the topic, *On Caring* (New York: Harper & Row, 1971). Like all theory, Mayeroff's work has its limitations. For example, his writing predates sensitivity to gender-excluding language, and he was not aware of the strides being made in working with people with developmental handicaps, which make them capable of the growth he seems to deny them. His concepts and analysis, however, have a depth that allows their use in understanding different caring perspectives.

2. Throughout the book, we quote several people from a variety of caregiving settings, both formal and informal, interviewed as part of a study conducted by the Rosalynn Carter Institute (Nottingham et al. 1993). The authors of that study were not in a position to verify whether those interviewed met the criteria of caring we are developing here with Mayeroff's help; however, we quote from their responses where their words suggest the existence of some dimensions of the ideal of caregiving that we are advancing.

CHAPTER 3

1. Although this section is addressed primarily to formal (professional) caregivers in their relationships to clients, many of the points are applicable, with some translation and interpretation, to the realm of informal (lay) caregiving.

2. These two professional roles should not be understood as a mutually exclusive dichotomy. As Schön developed his analysis of modes of professional action, he contrasted technical rationality, the expert mode, with a radically negative view (he did not label this position) of professionals that denied the legitimacy of any of their expertise. Reflective practice is, in effect, a synthesis of radically positive and radically negative views of the role of the expert.

3. Informal (lay) caregivers are also often in a position of power relative to those for whom they care.

4. As with technical rationality and reflective practice, these two forms of power are not mutually exclusive. Human beings, by virtue of their imperfection, always exercise some mixture of directive and synergic power.
5. These notions may apply to informal caregivers as well.

CHAPTER 4

1. We use *services* here as a singular term to refer to whatever is provided to the recipient on the right-hand side of the transaction. This typically includes both formal services and informal supports.
2. See Biegel, Sales, and Schulz (1991) for a thorough discussion of how different illnesses determine service needs differently, and Singer and Irvin (1989) for a detailed listing of services offered in family-support programs in seventeen states.

References

Agranoff, R. 1977. Services integration. In *Managing human services*, edited by W. F. Anderson, B. J. Frieden, and M. J. Murphy. Washington, D.C.: International City Management Association.

Aldrich, F.; A. Holliday; J. Colwell; B. Johnson; E. Smith; and R. Sharpley. 1971. The mental retardation service delivery system project: A survey of mental retardation service usage and needs among families with retarded children in selected areas of Washington state. *Research report.* Vol. 1. Olympia, Wash.: Office of Research.

American Association of Retired Persons, and Travelers Companies Foundation. 1988. *National survey of caregivers: Summary of findings.* Washington, D.C.: American Association of Retired Persons, and Travelers Companies Foundation.

Anderson, R., and J. F. Newman. 1973. Societal and individual determinants of medical care utilization in the United States. *Millbank Memorial Fund Quarterly* 51:95–124.

Avison, W. R.; R. J. Turner; S. Noh; and K. N. Speechler. 1993. The impact of caregiving: Comparisons of different family contexts and experiences. In *Caregiving systems: Formal and informal helpers,* edited by S. H. Zarit, L. I. Pearlin, and K. W. Shaie. Hillsdale, N.J.: Lawrence Erlbaum.

Bakan, D. 1966. *The duality of human existence: An essay on psychology and religion.* Chicago: Rand McNally.

Baldwin, S. 1985. *The costs of caring.* London: Routledge.

Bass, D. M., and L. S. Noelker. 1987. The influence of family caregivers on elders' use of in-home services: An expanded conceptual framework. *Journal of Health and Social Behavior* 28:184–96.

Bayley, M. 1973. *Mental handicap and community care.* London: Routledge.

Biegel, D.; E. Sales; and R. Schulz. 1991. *Family caregiving in chronic illness.* Newbury Park, Calif.: Sage.

Bone, M.; B. Spain; and F. Martin. 1972. *Plans and provisions for the mentally handicapped.* London: Allen and Unwin.

Browning, D. S. 1973. *Generative man: Psychoanalytic perspectives.* Philadelphia: Westminster Press.

Buber, M. 1958. *I and thou.* 2d ed. New York: Scribners.

Burland, J. 1992. The right to treatment. *Alliance for the Mentally Ill of Vermont Newsletter,* no. 23.

Caserta, M. S.; D. A. Lund; S. D. Wright; and D. E. Redburn. 1987. Caregivers to dementia patients: The utilization of community services. *Gerontologist* 27: 209–14.

Chetwynd, J. 1985. Factors contributing to stress on mothers caring for an intellectually handicapped child. *British Journal of Social Work* 15:295–304.

Coll, B. 1973. *Perspectives in public welfare: A history.* Washington, D.C.: U.S. Department of Health, Education, and Welfare. U.S. Government Printing Office.

Coyne, A. C. 1991. Information and referral service usage among caregivers for dementia patients. *Gerontologist* 31:384–88.

Craig, J. H., and M. Craig. 1973. *Synergic power: Beyond domination and submissiveness.* Berkeley, Calif.: Proactive Press.

Cross, T. C. 1989. *Towards a culturally competent system of care.* Washington, D.C.: CASSP Technical Assistance Center, Georgetown University.

Daniels, P. K., and C. A. Schwartz, eds. 1994. *Encyclopedia of Associations.* Detroit: Gale Research.

Demos, J. 1983. Family home care: Historical notes and reflections. In *Family home care: Critical issues for services and policies,* edited by R. Perlman. New York: Haworth Press.

DHHS. 1995. *Performance measurement in selected public health programs.* Washington, D.C.: Public Health Service.

Dokecki, P. R. 1983. The place of values in the world of psychology and public policy. *Peabody Journal of Education* 60 (3): 108–25.

Dunlap, W. 1976. Services for families of the developmentally disabled. *Social Work* 21:220–23.

Dunst, C. J.; C. M. Trivette; and A. G. Deal. 1988. *Enabling and empowering families.* Cambridge, Mass.: Brookline Books.

Edwards, R. L. 1990. Professional and family caregivers: A social work perspective. In *The professional and family caregiver: Dilemmas, rewards, and new directions,* edited by J. Nottingham and J. Nottingham. Americus: Rosalynn Carter Institute, Georgia Southwestern State University.

Eggers, W., and R. Ng. 1993. *Social and health service privatization: A survey of state and county governments.* Los Angeles: Reason Foundation.

Erikson, E. H. 1967. *Insight and responsibility.* New York: Norton.

Farber, B. 1975. Family adaptation to severely mentally retarded children. In *The mentally retarded and society: A social science perspective,* edited by M. Begab and S. Richardson. Baltimore: University Park Press.

Foege, W. H. 1993. Preventive medicine and public health. *Journal of the American Medical Association* 270 (2): 251–52.

Forrester, J. 1982. Planning in the face of power. *Journal of the American Planning Association* 48:67–80.

———. 1983. Critical theory and organizational analysis. In *Beyond method: Strategies for social research,* edited by G. Morgan. Beverly Hills: Sage.

Fox, K. A. 1974. *Social indicators and social theory: Elements of an operational system.* New York: Wiley.

Freudenberger, H. J. 1990. Caring for the caregiver: Recognizing and dealing with burnout. In *The professional and family caregiver: Dilemmas, rewards, and new directions,* edited by J. Nottingham and J. Nottingham. Americus: Rosalynn Carter Institute, Georgia Southwestern State University.

Garrard, S. B., and J. B. Richmond. 1963. Psychological aspects of the management of chronic diseases and handicapping conditions in childhood. In *The psychological basis of medical practice,* edited by H. Lief, V. Lief, and N. Lief. New York: Harper & Row.

Gilbert, N. 1973. Assessing service delivery models: Some unsettled questions. *Welfare in Review* 10 (3): 25–33.

Glendinning, C. 1983. *Unshared care.* London: Allen and Unwin.

Goldfarb, L. A.; M. J. Brotherson; J. A. Summers; and A. P. Turnbull. 1986. *Meeting the challenge of disability or chronic illness: A family guide.* Baltimore: Paul H. Brookes.

Goode, W. 1975. *World revolution and family patterns.* Glencoe, Ill.: Free Press.

Gottleib, J. 1975. Public, peer, and professional attitudes toward mentally retarded persons. In *The mentally retarded and society: A social science perspective,* edited by M. Begab and S. Richardson. Baltimore: University Park Press.

Graham, H. 1983. Caring: A labour of love. In *A Labour of love,* edited by J. Finch and D. Groves. London: Routledge.

Gray, D. P. 1990. The challenge of caring for the chronically mentally ill. In *The professional and family caregiver: Dilemmas, rewards, and new directions,* edited by J. Nottingham and J. Nottingham. Americus: Rosalynn Carter Institute, Georgia Southwestern State University.

Gronbjerg, K. 1990. Poverty and nonprofit organizational behavior. *Social Service Review* 62 (2): 208–43.

Groves, I. D. 1994. *R.C. v. Hornsby consent decree: Performance and outcome review.* Tampa: Florida Mental Health Institute.

Habermas, J. 1971. *Knowledge and the human interest.* Boston: Beacon Press.

———. 1973. *Theory and practice.* Boston: Beacon Press.

———. 1975. *Legitimation crisis.* Boston: Beacon Press.

Hay, D., and D. Oken. 1977. The psychological stresses of ICU nursing. In *Coping with physical illness,* edited by R. H. Moos. New York: Plenum.

Hetherington, E. M.; M. Cox; and R. Cox. 1977. The development of children in mother headed families. Paper presented at the Families in Contemporary America Conference, George Washington University, Washington, D.C., June 11, 1977.

Hewett, S. 1972. *The family and the handicapped child.* London: Allen and Unwin.

Hill, R. 1949. *Families under stress.* New York: Harper.

Hirst, M. A. 1992. Employment patterns of mothers with a disabled young person. *Work, Employment, and Society* 6 (1): 87–101.

Hobbs, N.; P. R. Dokecki; K. V. Hoover-Dempsey; R. M. Moroney; M. W. Shayne; and K. H. Weeks. 1984. *Strengthening families.* San Francisco: Jossey-Bass.

Hodge, M. C. 1992. Outpatient commitment: Beginning a dialogue. *National Association of Case Management* 1 (5): 1–5.

Hooyman, N. 1995. *Feminist perspectives on family care: Policies for gender justice.* Thousand Oaks, Calif.: Sage.

Imre, R. W. 1982. *Knowing and caring.* New York: University Press of America.

Institute of Medicine. 1994. *Reducing risks for mental disorders: Frontiers for preventive intervention research.* Edited by P. J. Mrazek and R. J. Haggerty. Washington, D.C.: National Academy Press.

Joseph, K. 1974. Britain: A decadent utopia. *Guardian* (October): 21.

Joshi, H. 1987. The cost of caring. In *Women and poverty,* edited by C. Glendinning and J. Millar. Brighton: Wheatsheaf Books.

Justice, R.; J. Bradley; and G. O'Connor. 1971. Foster family care for the retarded: Management concerns for the caretaker. *Mental Retardation* 9 (4): 12–15.

Kagan, S.; D. Powell; B. Weissbourd; and E. Zigler, eds. 1987. *America's family support programs.* New Haven: Yale University Press.

Kagan, S., and B. Weissbourd. 1994. *Putting families first: America's family support movement and the challenge of change.* San Francisco: Jossey-Bass.

Kaiser Permanente and Andersen Consulting, SC. 1993. *1993 Quality Report Card.* Oakland, Calif.: Kaiser Permanente.

Kane, R. A., and J. D. Penrod. 1993. Family caregiving policies: Insights from an intensive longitudinal study. In *Caregiving systems: Formal and informal helpers,* edited by S. H. Zarit, L. I. Pearlin, and K. W. Shaie. Hillsdale, N.J.: Lawrence Erlbaum.

Kelly, J. G. 1990. Changing contexts and the field of community psychology. *American Journal of Community Psychology* 18:769–92.

Kettner, P., and L. Martin. 1996. The impact of declining resources and purchasing of service contracting on private non-profit agencies. *Administration in Social Work* 20 (3): 21–38.

Kettner, P.; R. Moroney; and L. Martin. 1990. *Designing and managing programs.* Newbury Park, Calif.: Sage.

Land, H., and H. Rose. 1985. Compulsory altruism for some or an altruistic society for all. In *In defence of welfare,* edited by P. Bean, J. Ferris, and D. Whynes. London: Tavistock.

Lansky, D. 1993. The new responsibility: Measuring and reporting on quality. *Joint Commission Journal on Quality Improvement* 19:545–51.

Lasch, C. 1978. *Haven in a heartless world: The family besieged.* New York: Basic Books.

Laslett, P. 1965. *The world we have lost.* London: Methuen.

Lawton, M. P.; E. M. Brody; A. Saperstein; and M. Grimes. 1989. Respite services for caregivers: Research findings for service planning. *Home Health Care Services Quarterly* 10 (1–2): 5–32.

Lazarus, R. S., and S. Folkman. 1984. *Stress, appraisal, and coping.* New York: Springer.

Lebacqz, K. 1985. *Professional ethics: Power and paradox.* Nashville: Abingdon Press.

Leira, A. 1994. Concepts of caring: Loving, thinking, and doing. *Social Service Review* 68 (2): 185–201.

Links Letter. 1994. Washington, D.C.: Links at Bazelon Center for Mental Health Law.

Locke, D. 1992. *Increasing multicultural understanding: A comprehensive model.* Newbury Park, Calif.: Sage.

Manderscheid, R. 1994. *Mental health statistical improvement program: Mental health component of a health plan report card: Progress report.* Rockville, Md.: Center for Mental Health Services.

Manderscheid, R., and M. Sonnerschein. 1992. *Mental health: United States.* Rockville, Md.: USDHHS, Center for Mental Health Services, and National Institute for Mental Health.

Marshner, C. 1981. The pro-family movement and traditional values. In *What is pro family policy?,* edited by L. Kagan. New Haven: Yale University Press.

Martin, J., and A. White. 1988. *The financial circumstances of disabled adults living in private households.* London: HMSO.

Maslach, C., and S. E. Jackson. 1981. The measurement of experienced burnout. *Journal of Occupational Behavior* 2:99–113.

Matthews, A. M. 1993. Issues in the examination of the caregiving relationship. In *Caregiving systems: Formal and informal helpers,* edited by S. H. Zarit, L. I. Pearlin, and K. W. Shaie. Hillsdale, N.J.: Lawrence Erlbaum.

Mayeroff, M. 1971. *On caring.* New York: Harper & Row.

McCubbin, H. I., and J. Patterson. 1983. The family stress process: The double ABCX model of adjustment and adaptation. In *Social stress and the family: Advances and developments in family stress theory and research,* edited by

H. I. McCubbin, M. B. Sussman, and J. M. Patterson. New York: Haworth.

McGinnis, J. M., and W. H. Foege. 1993. Actual causes of death in the United States. *Journal of the American Medical Association* 270 (18): 2207–12.

McMurtry, S.; E. Netting; and P. Kettner. 1990. "How non-profits adapt to a stringent environment." *Nonprofit Management and Leadership* 1 (3): 235–52.

McPheeters, H. L. 1990. The professional and family caregiver: Medical/psychiatric issues. In *The professional and family caregiver: Dilemmas, rewards, and new directions,* edited by J. Nottingham and J. Nottingham. Americus: Rosalynn Carter Institute, Georgia Southwestern State University.

Miller, B. 1993. Congregations increase charitable work even as donations show a decline. *Chronicle of Philanthropy* 7:7–8, 15–17.

Minnesota Department of Human Services. 1988. *Caregivers need care too: Final report.* St. Paul, Minn.: Adult Services Section, Division of Community Services.

Moroney, R. M. 1991. *Social policy and social work: Critical essays on the welfare state.* Hawthorne, N.Y.: Aldine.

———. 1986. *Shared responsibility: Families and social policy.* Hawthorne, N.Y.: Aldine.

———. 1977. Needs assessment for human services. In *Managing human services,* edited by W. F. Anderson, B. J. Frieden, and M. J. Murphy. Washington, D.C.: International City Management Association.

Moroney, R. M., and P. R. Dokecki. 1984. The family and the professions: Implications for public policy. *Journal of Family Issues* 5:224–38.

Mullan, J. T. 1993. Barriers to the use of formal services among Alzheimer's caregivers. In *Caregiving systems: Formal and informal helpers,* edited by S. H. Zarit, L. I. Pearlin, and K. W. Shaie. Hillsdale, N.J.: Lawrence Erlbaum.

National Center for Health Statistics. 1993. *Healthy People 2000 Review, 1992.* Hyattsville, Md.: Public Health Service.

National Center for Service Integration. 1993. *Going to scale with a comprehensive services agenda: Summary of a Wingspread conference.* Falls Church, Va.: National Center for Services Integration.

National Committee for Quality Assurance. 1993. *Health employer data and information set (HEDIS) 2.0.* Washington, D.C.: National Committee for Quality Assurance.

Newman, S. 1976. *Housing adjustments of older people.* Ann Arbor: Institute of Social Research, University of Michigan.

Noelker, L. S., and D. M. Bass. 1989. Home care for elderly persons: Linkages between formal and informal caregivers. *Journal of Gerontology* 44:563–70.

Nottingham, J. A.; D. Haigler; D. L. Smith; and P. Davis. 1993. *Caregivers and caregiving in West Central Georgia.* Americus: Rosalynn Carter Institute, Georgia Southwestern State University.

Nottingham, J., and J. Nottingham, eds. 1990. *The professional and family care-*

giver: Dilemmas, rewards, and new directions. Americus: Rosalynn Carter Institute, Georgia Southwestern State University.

Osborne, D., and T. Gaebler. 1992. *Reinventing government.* New York: Plume.

Parker, G. 1992. *With this body: Caring and disability in marriage.* Buckingham, England: Open University Press.

Parker, R. 1981. Tending and social policy. In *A new look at the personal social services,* edited by E. Goldberg and S. Hatch. London: Policy Studies Institute.

Perring, C.; J. Twigg; and K. Atkin. 1990. *Families caring for people diagnosed as mentally ill: The literature reexamined.* London: HMSO.

Pilisuk, M., and S. H. Parks. 1988. Caregiving: Where families need help. *Social Work* 33:436–40.

Pines, M. 1994. *Family investment strategies: Improving the lives of children and communities.* Washington, D.C.: Partners for Livable Places.

Poulshock, S. W., and G. T. Deimling. 1984. Families caring for elders in residence: Issues in the measurement of burden. *Journal of Gerontology* 39:230–39.

Prigerson, H. G. 1991. Determinants of hospice utilization among terminally ill geriatric patients. *Home Health Care Services Quarterly* 12 (4): 81–111.

Quine, L., and J. Pahl. 1985. Examining the causes of stress in families with severely mentally handicapped children. *British Journal of Social Work* 15:501–17.

Rein, M. 1970. Cd. 272 Social policy: Issues of choice and change. New York: Random House.

Report of the poor law commission of 1832. 8, 1905.

Richardson, E. 1973. Services integration: Next steps. Secretarial Memorandum, June 1, 1973. Cited in Marshall Kaplan. 1973. *Integration of human services in HEW: An evaluation of service integration projects.* Washington, D.C.: DHEW, SRS.

Richmond, J. B. 1973. The family and the handicapped child. *Clinical Proceedings, Children's Hospital National Medical Center* 29:156–64.

Riley, L., and S. Nagi, eds. 1980. *Disability in the United States: A compendium of data on prevalence and programs.* Columbus: Ohio State University.

Rosenbaum, E. 1988. *A taste of my own medicine.* New York: Random House.

Russell, L. B. 1993. The role of prevention in health reform. *New England Journal of Medicine* 329 (5): 352–54.

Sainsbury, P., and J. Grad de Alarcon. 1971. The psychiatrist and the geriatric patient: The effects of community care on the family of the geriatric patient. *Journal of Geriatric Psychiatry* 4 (1): 23–41.

Sarason, S. B. 1985. *Caring and compassion in clinical practice.* San Francisco: Jossey-Bass.

Schön, D. 1983. *The reflective practitioner.* New York: Basic Books.

Schorr, A. 1968. Beyond pluck and luck. *Explorations in social policy.* New York: Basic Books.

Schorr, A., and P. Moen. 1977. Single parents: Public and private image. Paper presented for the Task Force on Mental Health and the Family. President's Commission on Mental Health.

Schottland, C. 1963. *The social security programs in the United States.* New York: Appleton-Century-Crofts.

Schreiber, L. 1993. The cure for doctors. *Lelle* 101 (2): 146–49.

Sheehan, N. 1988. *The caregiver information project: Establishing an information network for family caregivers.* Storrs, Conn.: Department of Aging, State of Connecticut.

Sines, D., and J. Bicknell. 1985. *Caring for mentally handicapped people in the community.* London: Harper & Row.

Singer, G. H. S., and L. K. Irvin. 1989. Family caregiving, stress, and support. In *Support for caregiving families: Enabling positive adaptation to disability,* edited by G. H. S. Singer and L. K. Irvin. Baltimore: Paul H. Brookes.

Smyth, M., and N. Robus. 1989. *The financial circumstances of families with disabled children living in private households.* London: HMSO.

Sokoly, M. M., and P. R. Dokecki. 1992. Ethical perspectives on family-centered early intervention. *Infants and Young Children* 4 (4): 23–32.

Sorokin, P. 1946. *The crisis of our age.* New York: Dutton.

Stephens, M. A. P. 1993. Understanding barriers to caregiver's use of formal services: The caregiver's perspective. In *Caregiving systems: Formal and informal helpers,* edited by S. H. Zarit, L. I. Pearlin, and K. W. Shaie. Hillsdale, N.J.: Lawrence Erlbaum.

Stone, R.; G. L. Cafferata; and J. Sangl. 1987. Caregivers of the frail elderly: A national profile. *Gerontologist* 27:616–26.

Sultz, H.; E. Schlesinger; W. Mosher; and J. Feldman. 1972. *Long-term childhood illness.* Pittsburgh: University of Pittsburgh Press.

Twigg, J. 1989. Not taking the strain. *Community Care* 27:16–18.

———. 1992. *Carers: Research and practice.* London: HMSO.

Twigg, J., and K. Atkin. 1993. *Policy and practice in informal care.* Buckingham, England: Open University Press.

Twigg, J.; K. Atkin; and C. Perring. 1990. *Carers and services: A review of research.* London: HMSO.

Ungerson, C. 1987. *Policy is personal: Sex, gender and informal care.* London: Tavistock.

———. 1990. The language of care: Crossing the boundaries. In *Gender and caring: Work and welfare in Britain and Scandinavia,* edited by C. Ungerson. London: Harvester/Wheatsheaf.

United States General Accounting Office. 1988. *Long-term care for the elderly: Issues of need, access, and cost.* Report to the Chairman, Subcommittee on Health and Long-Term Care, Select Committee on Aging, House of Representatives. Washington, D.C.: U.S. Government Printing Office.

Walker, B. 1989. Strategies for improving parent-professional cooperation. In *Support for caregiving families: Enabling positive adaptation to disability*, edited by G. H. S. Singer and L. K. Irvin. Baltimore: Paul H. Brookes.

White House Domestic Policy Council. 1993. *The President's Health Security Plan*. New York: Random House.

Wilkin, D. 1979. *Caring for the mentally handicapped child*. London: Groom Helm.

Wilson, E. 1977. *Women and the welfare state*. London: Tavistock.

Wuthnow, R. 1994. *Sharing the journey: Support groups and America's new quest for community*. New York: Free Press.

Yankelovich, Skelly, and White, Inc. 1977. *Raising children in a changing society*. Minneapolis: General Mills American Family Report.

Zarit, S. H., and L. I. Pearlin. 1993. Family caregiving: Integrating informal and formal systems for care. In *Caregiving systems: Formal and informal helpers*, edited by S. H. Zarit, L. I. Pearlin, and K. W. Shaie. Hillsdale, N.J.: Lawrence Erlbaum.

Zimmerman, D. L. 1994. Grading the graders: Using "report cards" to enhance the quality of care under health care reform. Issue Brief/No. 642. Washington, D.C.: National Health Policy Forum.

Annotated Bibliography

Resources for Formal (Professional)
and Informal (Family/Lay) Caregivers

Table of Contents

Garfield, Charles. 1995. *Sometimes my heart goes numb: Love and caregiving in a time of AIDS.* San Francisco: Jossey-Bass (298 pp.).

This book offers portraits of twenty caregivers of persons with HIV/AIDS. It also reveals the risks and rewards of giving care to a person with a chronic or life-threatening illness. Some of the topics discussed are active listening; coping with losses; bereavement; saying the right thing; and taking care of oneself while giving care to others.

Landau-Stanton, Judith. 1993. *AIDS, health, and mental health.* New York: Brunner/Mazel (343 pp.).

The authors of this book are concerned with assisting professionals to become better educated concerning the AIDS virus. Discussions include correcting AIDS myths, systems impacted by AIDS, populations at risk, health care providers at risk, and clinical management of AIDS.

ALZHEIMER'S DISEASE AND RELATED DISORDERS

Bridges, Barbara J. 1995. *Therapeutic caregiving: A practical guide for caregivers of persons with Alzheimer's and other dementia causing diseases.* Mill Creek, Wash.: BJB Publishing (214 pp.).

Therapeutic Caregiving offers professional expertise and practical advice. The author presents techniques for keeping people with dementia more functional physically and mentally. How to maintain adequate nutrition and oral hygiene, assist with bathing and dressing, help with exercise, manage behavior problems, and deal with confusion and depression are only some of the topics covered. Both long-term care professionals and family members can benefit from the practical suggestions and pictured exercises. Caregivers dealing with people who have strokes, Parkinson's disease, and so on would also benefit from this manual.

Coughlan, Patricia B. 1993. *Facing Alzheimer's: Family caregivers speak.* New York: Ballantine Books (261 pp.).

When the body and mind of a loved one begin to fail, the burden that falls on the caregiver can be overwhelming. In this deeply practical and warmhearted book, eight women who lived through their husbands' declines talk frankly about how they faced the agonizing decisions they had to make and live with, including acknowledging the illness, adjusting to profound changes in one's spouse, coping with crisis, nurturing one's own sanity and health, and preparing for the end and a new beginning.

Danforth, Art. 1984. *Living with Alzheimer's: Ruth's story.* Falls Church, Va.: Prestige Press (219 pp.).

Living with Alzheimer's: Ruth's Story is the moving and heartwarming story of the life shared by two victims of dementia: Art's wife, Ruth, whose mental deterioration he lived with every day for seven years, and Art, the caregiver. Art shares with the reader not only his love for Ruth and his fears for her safety but also his anger and sense of guilt.

Doernberg, Myrna. 1986. *Stolen mind: The slow disappearance of Ray Doernberg.* Chapel Hill, N.C.: Algonquin Books (223 pp.).

A wife vividly tells the story of her husband's progressive dementia; what she, her husband, and their two sons experienced dealing with his disease; and the many ways this disaster affected their family.

Dwyer, Sharon A. R.; Phillip D. Sloane; and Ann Louise Barrick. 1995. *Solving bathing problems in persons with Alzheimer's disease and related dementias: A training and reference manual for caregivers.* Chapel Hill: University of North Carolina (68 pp.).

The authors provide answers to commonly asked questions about problems related to bathing persons with dementia. General guidelines for bathing persons with dementia and procedures for dealing with specific bathing problems are included. Also explained are methods for developing a personal hygiene care plan and maintaining the quality of bathing procedures.

Feil, Naomi. 1993. *The validation breakthrough: Simple techniques for communicating with people with "Alzheimer's-type dementia."* Baltimore: Health Professions Press (320 pp.).

Validation therapy is a tool to aid in communication with people who have Alzheimer's-type dementia. It shows caregivers how they can reduce conflict and stress by validating feelings rather than focusing on confusion. The author explains specifically how to use validation therapy with individuals who are maloriented, time confused, repetitive movers, and so on.

Gruetzner, Howard. 1992. *Alzheimer's: A caregiver's guide and sourcebook.* New York: John Wiley & Sons (310 pp.).

This guide leads the reader through the realities of caring for and coping with a person with Alzheimer's disease. The latest developments in treatment and care options are detailed. Topics covered include the symptoms and traits of Alzheimer's, what to expect at each progressive stage, how to respond to behavior problems, the full range of treatments and supportive services available, suggestions on managing personal stress, the importance of the family in the successful care of Alzheimer's patients, and ways to understand feelings and the impact of grief. The author shows caregivers how to make the care they give more rewarding and more effective and the life of the patient safer and more comfortable.

Heston, Leonard L., and June A. White. 1991. *The vanishing mind: A practical guide to Alzheimer's disease and other dementias.* New York: W. H. Freeman (191 pp.).

The authors of this guide offer specific and detailed information on dementia and various diseases that result in a condition of dementia. Chapters explore topics including signs and symptoms of dementia, diseases that cause dementia, specialists and tests, medical treatment and management of dementia, care alternatives, and practical matters such as children, neighbors, finances, and insurance.

Mace, Nancy L. 1990. *Dementia care: Patient, family, and community.* Baltimore: Johns Hopkins University Press (400 pp.).

This sourcebook covers a wealth of information on dementia care, including the diagnostic assessment of patients, their clinical care, management of behavior problems, therapeutic activity, and issues in late-stage care. The family is considered in discussions of support, home environment, respite care, and financial and legal considerations. Long-term care services, volunteer programs, residential care, and public policy are explored.

Murphy, Beverly Bigtree. 1995. *He used to be somebody: A journey into Alzheimer's disease through the eyes of a caregiver.* Boulder: Gibbs Associates (348 pp.).

This author gives a firsthand account of the onset of Alzheimer's disease through its progression into the final stages. Murphy has a unique view of this illness from professional and personal standpoints, resulting in her ability to offer practical insights on subjects such as adapting the home, handling incontinence, dealing with the behavior changes, and grief and mourning. The author/caregiver shares the sense of isolation, fear, loss, and continuous state of mourning one goes through when losing a loved one to a progressive, degenerative disease. A special feature of this book is the inclusion of the reprinted words of famous songs that poignantly illustrate the significant stages of Alzheimer's disease and the feelings of the people involved with the illness during each of these stages.

Roberts, D. Jeanne. 1991. *Taking care of caregivers: For families and others who care for people with Alzheimer's disease and other forms of dementia.* Palo Alto, Calif.: Bull Publishing (181 pp.).

Taking Care of Caregivers inspires and empowers caregivers so that they can maintain their own health, happiness, and sanity in order to provide loving care for the person who is ill. With descriptions of the problems and exercises to help find solutions, this guide covers many important topics, including the needs of caregivers, communication and feelings, grief and its various phases, sharing and support, and stress management techniques.

Wright, Lore K. 1993. *Alzheimer's disease and marriage: An intimate account.* Newbury Park, Calif.: Sage (147 pp.).

Alzheimer's Disease and Marriage peers into caregiving research and personal data on individual relationships to uncover the profound effects of Alzheimer's disease on marriage. The author shows how the disease invades various dimensions of marriage and how spouses retain or lose awareness of each other.

Among the marital dimensions explored are day-to-day aspects of a relationship, such as household tasks, tension, companionship, affection and sexuality, and commitment. Clinical assessment strategies and guidelines for interventions are described. Details on how to approach and interact with an affected spouse are also provided.

BOOKS FOR CHILDREN

Attention Deficit Hyperactivity Disorder

Quinn, Patricia O., and Judith M. Stern. 1991. *Putting on the brakes: Young people's guide to understanding attention deficit hyperactivity disorder.* New York: Magination Press (226 pp.).

This down-to-earth, upbeat guide contains a wealth of information and practical suggestions for coping with the problems that attention deficit hyperactivity disorder (ADHD) presents. The authors explore the nature and treatment of ADHD, as well as gaining control, getting support, and making friends. Quinn and Stern's purpose is to give children a sense of control and a perception of obtainable goals.

Wodrich, David L. 1994. *Attention deficit hyperactivity disorder: What every parent wants to know.* Baltimore: Paul H. Brookes (291 pp.).

Through detailed explanations, helpful checklists, and case examples, this book combines Wodrich's professional expertise with a personal sensitivity developed from working closely with the families of children with attention deficit hyperactivity disorder. This book will help prepare parents with children suffering from ADHD for the challenges facing them at home and school and for the many decisions they will have to make about intervention and education.

Cancer

Trillin, Alice. 1996. *Dear Bruno.* New York: New Press (32 pp.).

This book is written for children who have cancer (or other serious illnesses) by a woman who previously had cancer and recovered. It is written as a letter that discusses the ill person's experiences with physicians and hospitals and what it is like to have a serious illness. This book is nicely illustrated by Edward Koren and has a foreword by Paul Newman.

Cerebral Palsy

Grimm, Eric. N.d. *Walk with me.* Washington, D.C.: United Cerebral Palsy Association (50 pp.).

Walk with Me is a touching story, written by an eight-year-old boy with cerebral palsy. In it, Eric tells what it is like to be a child facing this disability and describes the feelings that he experiences. Included is a checklist of strategies to use when communicating with a person who has a disability. This book is excellent reading for children who interact with a child with cerebral palsy, either at school or at home.

Diabetes

Mulder, Linnea. 1992. *Sarah and Puffle: A story for children about diabetes.* New York: Magination Press (29 pp.).
A stuffed sheep comes to life just in time to help a young girl who is feeling angry and sad because she has diabetes. Puffle's funny rhymes are full of valuable advice sure to comfort all children with diabetes and to further understanding by siblings and friends. Parents will appreciate the clearly written introduction.

Down's Syndrome

Berkus, Clara W. 1992. *Charlsie's chuckle.* Rockville, Md.: Woodbine House (32 pp.).
This is the story of an adventurous seven-year-old boy with Down's syndrome who becomes the local hero when his laugh brings harmony to his hometown. On his birthday, Charlsie gets a bicycle and takes off on a special adventure. This book teaches that every child can make a significant contribution and that a little laughter can make a big difference.

Epilepsy

Moss, Deborah M. 1989. *Lee: The rabbit with epilepsy.* Kensington, Md.: Woodbine House (12 pp.).
The imaginative tale of Lee and her family explains epilepsy in a manner that children can easily understand. Lee's epilepsy is followed from her first seizure through her diagnosis and treatment. The author takes a compassionate yet realistic view of epilepsy. The book is a valuable guide for an epileptic child as well as the sibling or friend of one. The message is one of hope and understanding regarding children with disabilities.

General Topics

Kriegsman, Kay H.; Elinor L. Zaslow; and Jennifer O'Zmura-Rechsteiner. 1992. *Taking charge: Teenagers talk about life and physical disabilities.* Rockville, Md.: Woodbine House (164 pp.).

Taking Charge delivers honest advice on a wide range of issues that teens with physical disabilities face during adolescence. This book covers three major areas of concern: part 1 focuses on the individual and self-esteem; part 2 explores relationships with friends, family, and the community; and part 3 looks toward the future with a discussion of long- and short-term goals and how to achieve them. Appendixes include a wealth of useful information.

Peterken, Allan. 1993. *What about me?* New York: Magination Press (32 pp.).

When children become seriously ill, their brothers and sisters are often confused and experience conflicting emotions. Children will identify with Laura, a young girl with a sick brother, who experiences the normal feelings of confusion, guilt, anger, and isolation when her parents seem to spend all their time at the hospital and all the attention is focused on her ill brother. Children reading this story will see their feelings being acknowledged and can gain a greater understanding of their situation.

Powell, Thomas H., and Peggy A. Gallagher. 1993. *Brothers and sisters: A special part of exceptional families.* Baltimore: Paul H. Brookes (289 pp.).

Rich with personal testimonies, this compelling book shares the joys and sorrows so familiar to exceptional families. Siblings speak openly about the challenges they encounter in interactions with their brothers or sisters and discuss how these interactions affect them in all aspects of their lives. Brimming with practical advice, this guide also includes a list of thirty parental strategies and twenty sibling strategies suggested by a panel of siblings.

Thompson, Mary. 1992. *My brother, Matthew.* Rockville, Md.: Woodbine House (28 pp.).

Siblings of children with disabilities often have trouble adjusting and have feelings of being "left out." In this tale, David has a younger brother born with disabilities. He tells what happens in his family and what it is like to be Matthew's brother. Siblings' normal feelings of loneliness, rejection, and impatience are addressed, along with a message of hope and understanding.

Mental Illness

Lanskin, Pamela L., and Addie A. Moskowitz. 1991. *Wish upon a star: A story for children with a parent who is mentally ill.* New York: Magination Press (32 pp.).

Children of a parent with mental illness often feel confused, frightened, lonely, and ashamed. In this poignant tale, a little girl expresses her confusion over the behavior of her mentally ill mother and the hurt she feels when her mother doesn't seem to pay attention to her anymore. Children will be comforted by having their feelings described, and others will gain a greater appreciation for the difficulty these children face.

CANCER

Benjamin, Harold H. 1995. *The wellness community: Guide to fighting for recovery from cancer.* New York: G. P. Putnam's Sons (270 pp.).

This book contains many insightful ideas and a great deal of information about fighting for recovery from cancer. Topics include fighting for one's recovery; how to control stress; how to use directed visualization; how to regain hope, take back control, and reduce anger; common questions people with cancer ask; what the Wellness Community is and the services it provides; the Wellness Community nutrition guide; and a list of the Wellness Community facilities and additional resources.

Gee, Elizabeth D. 1992. *The light around the dark.* Hudson Street, N.Y.: National League for Nursing Press (150 pp.).

The Light around the Dark tells Elizabeth Gee's story of caring, of her life of living her ethics, and of her humanity. It tells a story of suffering and triumph, of despair and joys, and of accomplishments. In this work, anyone who has been touched by the complex experiences associated with cancer will be lifted up by the peace and strength she found throughout her life. Readers will be encouraged by her victorious struggles with living and dying, with being connected, being alone, mothering, spousing—in being all she could be.

Rosenblum, Daniel. 1993. *A time to hear, a time to help: Listening to people with cancer.* New York: Free Press (289 pp.).

Dr. Rosenblum, drawing on his long experience as a leading oncologist, shows that the greatest assistance friends, relatives, and even the physicians of people with cancer can offer is to treat them as full human beings with dignity and respect, rather than as "cancer patients." He points out that the most thoughtful and most comforting thing one can do many times is just to listen. *A Time to Hear, a Time to Help* is a personal testimony to the often difficult and painful process of learning how to listen. Through intimate portraits, Rosenblum teaches readers to understand the problems people with cancer and their caregivers face (anxiety, anger, denial, loss of self-esteem, facing death, and so on) and the importance of compassion, patience, and understanding in offering comfort to them.

CARE OF ELDERLY

Barresi, Charles M. 1993. *Ethnic elderly and long-term care.* New York: Springer (289 pp.).

Barresi gives a professional overview of the special needs of ethnic elderly persons. He explores ethnic variations in measurement of physical health; minority issues in family caregiving; black and Hispanic caregivers of dementia victims; self-care practices of black elders; institutional care in ethnic settings; models of ethnically sensitive care; and planning, policy, and practice.

Biegel, David E. 1990. *Aging and caregiving.* Newbury Park, Calif.: Sage (294 pp.). This book thoroughly covers research conducted in the area of aging and caregiving dealing with theory and methodology, cognitive and physical impairment, and public policy perspectives. Some of the specific topics covered are the psychological impact of caregiving on the caregiver; ethical issues in a family caregiving situation; stress of caregivers; and women as caregivers of the elderly.

Cantor, Marjorie H., ed. 1994. *Family caregiving: Agenda for the future.* San Francisco: American Society on Aging (149 pp.).

This book of readings contains papers presented at the 1993 Critical Issues Forum conducted by the American Society on Aging. Family caregiving is discussed from a number of angles, including research and personal perspectives, public policy agenda, and training with education. Also explored is the impact of social services and ethical, legal, and financial issues on caregivers.

Carlin, Vivian F., and Vivian E. Greenburg. 1992. *Should mom live with us?: And is happiness possible if she does?* New York: Lexington Books (195 pp.).

With rising costs of care, elderly people often find themselves dependent on their adult children for a place to live and for personal care. This guide is designed to help middle-aged children and their aging parents weigh all options and make good decisions about living together. With warmth and humor, the authors explore pros and cons, discuss alternatives, and then provide a blueprint for making it work.

Cohen, Donna, and Carl Eisdorfer. 1993. *Seven steps to effective parent care: A planning and action guide for adult children and their aging parents.* New York: G. P. Putnam's Sons (261 pp.).

Based on years of research and work with families, this book presents a coherent approach for caregiving that reframes aging and parent care as a process of problem solving to be managed by the entire family. The authors have segmented caregiving into small, easily accomplished steps and procedures that can substantially help in avoiding crises and family battles and eliminating many of the frustrations and fears that often accompany caring for an aging parent. Case histories are used to illustrate points. Complete listings of national and state agencies and social services involved in gerontology, mental health, and related areas are also included. Self-help exercises help readers evaluate their situations.

Decalmer, Peter, and Frank Glendenning, eds. 1993. *The mistreatment of elderly people.* Newbury Park, Calif.: Sage (192 pp.).

The Mistreatment of Elderly People argues for clearer explanations of elder abuse that go beyond immediate practical considerations and observations and gives clear guidelines for tackling and preventing the problem. The authors include discussions of key topics such as legal implications of abuse and neglect, issues for professionals dealing with elder abuse, approaches for dealing with abuse, and models for prevention of abuse.

Estes, Carroll L., and James H. Swan. 1993. *The long-term care crisis: Elders trapped in the no-care zone.* Newbury Park, Calif.: Sage (328 pp.).

The authors discuss the Prospective Payment System (PPS) for Medicare hospital reimbursement that was begun in 1984 and demonstrate its negative effects, especially on the elderly. They identify the failing of PPS and provide policy options to modify or replace it with a system that would foster greater equity in providing health care in America.

Fradkin, Louise G., and Angela Heath. 1992. *Caregiving of older adults.* Santa Barbara, Calif.: ABC-CLIO (250 pp.).

In *Caregiving of Older Adults,* readers will find information on types of caregivers and supports, financial and legal issues, safety and welfare, housing options, and nursing home placement. One chapter is dedicated to understanding the care receiver. Also included is a valuable list of resources.

Greenberg, Vivian E. 1989. *Your best is good enough: Aging parents and your emotions.* New York: Lexington Books (301 pp.).

Time-proven strategies for coping with the conflicts and stresses inherent in caring for elderly parents are provided. With insight and skill, Vivian Greenberg offers valuable information on the needs of the elderly, the vital role emotional involvement plays in caregiving, and the need for assertive and honest communication with one's parents. She explains how to realize and accept the limits of what one can do for his or her parents; how to determine unrealistic expectations; how to get brothers and sisters to share responsibilities; and how to cope with a difficult parent. Personal anecdotes and real-life cases make this compassionate guide important reading for those who must oversee the well-being of their parents while trying to preserve their own. An appendix containing information on available resources is included.

Greenberg, Vivian E. 1994. *Children of a certain age: Adults and their aging parents.* New York: Lexington Books (183 pp.).

In *Children of a Certain Age,* Greenberg reveals ways adult children and their aging parents can develop a mature, caring relationship based on mutual respect, trust, and friendship. She explains that parenthood is always in a state of change and growth and that parents who are open and responsive to their children not only learn from them but will feel rejuvenated rather than frustrated and left behind. This guide shows how this can be a time to change, heal old wounds, resolve conflicts, and touch each other with affection and understanding.

Gubrium, Jaber F. 1993. *Speaking of life: Horizons of meaning for nursing home residents.* Hawthorne, N.Y.: Aldine De Gruyter (197 pp.).

The author uses data drawn from interviews with long-term nursing home residents to explore the quality of their care and the resulting quality of their lives. These stories reveal to readers the diversity of people living in nursing homes, their views of family, their feelings of dependence/independence, their experiences of isolation and sense of self-esteem, and how they perceive the quality of their lives in nursing homes. The result is a wide variety of stories and information with valuable conceptual, methodological, and personal lessons.

Horn, Barbara J. 1990. *Facilitating self care practices in the elderly.* Binghamton, N.Y.: Haworth (185 pp.).

This professional guide covers several aspects of care practices in the elderly. Horn discusses medication regimens, compliance, adverse drug reactions, the Comprehensive Medication Assessment Interview guide, tailoring teaching to the elderly in home care, and family coping with caring for the elderly.

Kane, Rosalie A., and Joan D. Penrod, eds. 1995. *Family caregiving in an aging society: Policy perspectives.* Thousand Oaks, Calif.: Sage (202 pp.).

This book considers the ramifications of the U.S. caregiving policy, describing and evaluating many of the current services: respite care, individual and group therapy, and educational interventions. Topics include prospects for family caregiving, examining respite care, direct services for family caregivers, legal and ethical issues in family caregiving, and a caregiving policy for the aging family.

Kermis, Marguerite D. 1986. *Mental health in late life: The adaptive process.* Boston: Jones & Bartlett (392 pp.).

This volume offers a broad overview for providing appropriate and effective care for elderly persons experiencing emotional or cognitive distress. Kermis discusses the medical and ethical issues involved in caring for mentally frail elderly persons. Also provided is a discussion of programs and policies that have been advanced to deal with mental health needs of older people.

Koch, Tom. 1993. *A place in time: Care givers for their elderly.* Westport, Conn.: Praeger (236 pp.).

A Place in Time tells the personal stories of normal people who have chosen to care for their aging and fragile relatives at home. The author uses their stories to ask: What can we learn from the experiences of others? He provides vital and practical information for anyone considering physically caring for another. Appropriate for professional and lay readers.

Kosberg, Jordan I., ed. 1992. *Family care of the elderly: Social and cultural changes.* Newbury Park, Calif.: Sage (317 pp.).

The focus of this book is on family care of the elderly in sixteen different countries of the world, including the United States. Every author addressed each of the following areas in discussing elder care in his or her country: traditional characteristics of the country; societal changes occurring over time; consequences of societal changes; responses to the changes in the country; and future predictions for the care of the elderly by the family and by formal service systems in the country.

Levin, Nora Jean. 1993. *How to care for your parents: A handbook for adult children.* Friday Harbor, Wash.: Storm King Press (110 pp.).

This brief handbook tells readers what to expect in elder care. It includes information on the kind of decisions that will need to be made, on the practical and emotional pitfalls that can occur, and on how to juggle the sometimes conflicting obligations to oneself, one's family, and one's parents. The author uses a twenty-eight-step program including time management, finances, home safety, and how best to help seniors in need.

McGurn, Sheelagh. 1992. *Under one roof: Caring for an aging parent.* Park Ridge, Ill.: Parkside Publishing (174 pp.). [Now available for purchase from Under One Roof, P.O. Box 9131, Mt. Prospect, IL 60056.]

In this book, Sheelagh McGurn speaks to the increasing number of people in the "sandwich generation": those who are now taking care of both their young families and their aging parents. Many of these people are overwhelmed trying to fulfill effectively their roles as spouse, parent, and caregiver. Finding doctors, arranging home health care, and coping with loved ones whose physical, mental, and emotional health may be failing all add to the normal stresses of working and raising a family. Through personal experiences and interviews, McGurn addresses the day-to-day problems of caregivers and offers them both daily coping strategies and hope for the future.

Nelson-Morrill, Creston, ed. 1993. *Florida caregiver's handbook: An essential resource guide for caregivers and their older loved ones.* 2d ed. Tallahassee, Fla.: HealthTrac Books (272 pp.).

This handbook covers a wide range of topics important to caregivers, including the impact of caregiving on caregivers and their families and on caregivers employed outside the home, long-distance caregiving, loss and grief, dementia, medication management, changes that may occur in the elderly as part of the normal aging process, alcohol and substance abuse, legal considerations, financial planning, nursing home decisions, dealing with the system, Medicare and Medicaid, and advocating for the care receiver. An extensive listing of elder services and caregiver support organizations with addresses and phone numbers is included. (This manual is written especially for Florida, but much of the material is helpful to people living in other states.)

Ory, Marcia G., and Alfred P. Duncker, eds. 1992. *In-home care for older people: Health and supportive services.* Newbury Park, Calif.: Sage (214 pp.).

The purpose of this book is to summarize what is known about home care for the elderly and to identify a research agenda that highlights the use of in-home services for older people with different functional needs, the effectiveness of different types or packages of services for different populations, and the coordination of in-home services with traditional medical services. The focus is on older people in need of long-term care. The significant contribution made by family and friends and the burdens that families experience in providing care are recognized.

Pritchard, Jacki. 1992. *The abuse of elderly people: A handbook for professionals*. Philadelphia: Jessica Kingsley Publishers (174 pp.).

The Abuse of Elderly People is a resource and manual for the variety of professionals who work with elderly people. The four main aims of the book are to define elder abuse, to raise the consciousness about elder abuse, to develop skills in recognizing elder abuse, and to develop ways of dealing with elder abuse. The handbook provides a range of scenarios and exercises dealing with each of these areas.

Rob, Caroline. 1991. *The caregiver's guide: Helping elderly relatives cope with health and safety problems*. Boston: Houghton Mifflin (458 pp.).

Sensible, basic information is provided to assist in handling medical emergencies for the elderly, recognizing both physical and mental problems, working with the latest medical advances for chronic disorders, keeping elders independent longer, and locating social services. This book is for those who are stepping in to help an older relative or friend who can no longer grapple alone with medical problems and daily living arrangements. Every section of the book is full of accessible, up-to-the-minute information about physical and emotional health. The chapters of *The Caregiver's Guide* are organized by conditions common in older people. The final chapter is a useful guide to accessing the social service system and network of support in communities around the country.

Rogg, Carla S., and Oskar H. Rogg. 1995. *Georgia senior resource guide: A resource guide for older adults, caregivers, and eldercare professionals*. Atlanta: Care Solutions (258 pp.).

This resource guide was designed to answer many of the questions older adults, their caregivers, and professionals have about elder care and to help them make informed decisions about finding and using elder-care services. It provides basic information about elder-care services specific to Georgia. Chapter titles include "Aging in Place," "Housing Options," "Legal and Financial Aspects of Aging," "Health Insurance," "Health Care," "Caregiving," and "Resources." The "Resource" section lists more than 2,100 specific providers and the services they offer.

Safford, Florence, and George I. Krell, eds. 1992. *Gerontology for health profession-*

als: A practice guide. Washington, D.C.: National Association of Social Workers (NASW) (183 pp.).

> This book provides basic principles of a humanistic perspective in health care for all professionals, but its emphasis is on providing care for the elderly that recognizes humane values and asserts the dignity and worth of every care receiver. Topics include understanding the experience of aging; helping the incontinent; medication; differential assessment of dementia and depression; case management with the elderly; working with traditional and nontraditional families; ethical issues; death, bereavement, loss, and growth; and the impact of the elderly on the health care system with implications for the delivery of social services.

Salamon, Michael J., and Gloria Rosenthal. 1990. *Home or the nursing home: Making the right choices.* New York: Springer (112 pp.).

> The authors of this guide provide extensive information for caregivers trying to make the difficult decision between home care and nursing home care. Discussions include critical topics such as health care needs of elderly, life satisfaction, health care environments, bias/reality of nursing home versus home care, elders' and families' reactions to nursing home care, and guidelines for selecting a nursing home.

Silverstone, Barbara, and Helen K. Hyman. 1992. *Growing older together: A couple's guide to understanding and coping with the challenges of later life.* New York: Pantheon Books (344 pp.).

> This thoughtful and empathetic guide offers sensible, easy-to-follow advice on a variety of topics including the first signals of advancing age, retirement preparation, relationships between aging parents and their aging children, changing roles within a long-established relationship, and preserving autonomy when illness strikes. Also included are resource lists of supplementary reading, family service associations, and home-care agencies.

Smith, Kerri S. 1992. *Caring for your aging parents.* San Louis Obispo, Calif.: Impact Publishers (117 pp.).

> Working caregivers need a road map through the often confusing caregiving wilderness. *Caring for Your Aging Parents* provides just that. It gives quick and effective solutions to common caregiving concerns, including how to make your parents' home safer and more convenient; where to find free and low-cost help; how to reconcile work responsibilities with caregiving duties; how to put parents' legal and financial affairs in order; how to recognize potential medical problems; and how to regain your physical, mental, and emotional equilibrium.

Susik, D. Helen. 1995. *Hiring home caregivers: The family guide to in-home eldercare.* San Luis Obispo, Calif.: American Source Books (205 pp.).

This is an excellent resource guide for people who employ an in-home care helper. Topics include the role and cost of home caregivers, selecting and hiring, background checks, supervising a helper, dealing with taxes, insurance, laws, and agency-directed home care. The lengthy and helpful appendixes include tax information, publications, the IRS "tele-tax" information system, Eldercare locator, agencies on aging, and state organizations on aging.

Trieshmann, Roberta B. 1987. *Aging with a disability.* New York: Demos Publications (148 pp.).

This volume offers case studies and interviews on the topics of health, rehabilitation, and adjustment processes of older adults with disabilities. Discussion of the psychosocial and environmental impact of aging and methodological issues in aging and disability research offer valuable information for the professional interested in further research in this field.

Tuites, Ann. 1995. *From grandma with love.* Lancaster, Pa.: Starburst (158 pp.).

This small book offers practical, emotional, and spiritual support to people providing care to aging relatives. It aims to create peace, love, and harmony between the generations. With entries much like a journal, the author discusses such ideas as expectations, it's never too late to change, worrying about aging and dementia, encouragement, anger, relinquishing parental power, avoiding overprotection, and building self-esteem.

Young, Rosalie F. 1991. *Health, illness, and disability in later life.* Newbury Park, Calif.: Sage (183 pp.).

This book is a collection of essays dealing with health, illness, and disability. Essays cover topics such as status, behaviors, and risks of the elderly, health problems and family care, and the multidisciplinary aspects of health, illness, and disability in later life.

CARE OF TERMINALLY ILL

Sankar, Andrea. 1991. *Dying at home: A family guide for caregiving.* Baltimore: Johns Hopkins University Press (257 pp.).

This book, based on interviews with family members, professional caregivers, and care receivers, discusses the decision of whether to provide care at home for someone who is dying. The author believes the most important reason for dying at home is that it gives the people involved as much control as possible over the process of dying. Some of the topics discussed are preparing the home, maintaining communication with professional health care providers, maintaining the dignity of the person who is dying, financial resources, signs of approaching death, the funeral, hospice, ethical dilemmas, caregivers taking care of themselves, and grief.

CHILDREN WITH SPECIAL NEEDS

Autism

Hart, Charles A. 1993. *A parent's guide to autism: Answers to the most common questions.* New York: Pocket Books (244 pp.).

    Using a question-and-answer format, Hart presents information about autism and the people who have it. Included in the book is information on causes, symptoms, types of autism, diets, exercises, possible therapies and treatments, facilitated communication, and planning for the future. A resource list of books and organizations is also included.

Powers, Michael D. 1989. *Children with autism.* Rockville, Md.: Woodbine House (368 pp.).

    The autistic child appears to exist in an isolated world, impossible to reach. For a parent to overcome the fears such a condition naturally arouses, he or she needs a great deal of information and hope. Powers attempts to meet this need with this comprehensive guide. From a clear description of autism and its problems, treatments, and effect on the family to a discussion of legal rights, the author offers clear explanations with sensitivity and skill. The condition is explored from infancy to adulthood, including a discussion of residential programs and other options for adult autistics. A glossary of important terms, a reading list, and a resource guide are included.

Shulze, Craig B. 1993. *When snow turns to rain: One family's struggle to solve the riddle of autism.* Rockville, Md.: Woodbine House (216 pp.).

    When Snow Turns to Rain is a father's moving account of his family's experience with autism. Shulze recounts his personal struggle to accept and understand his son's autism and his determination to help his child through an array of treatment and educational programs. This book affirms the strength of the human spirit and attests to the needs of a family raising a child with a developmental disability.

Stehli, Annabel. 1991. *The sound of a miracle.* New York: Avon Books (241 pp.).

    The Sound of a Miracle is written by a mother who struggled to help her daughter, Georgie, who was diagnosed with autism. Stehli refused institutionalization as many experts and friends recommended, and she sought education and treatment for her child. A new treatment for autism—auditory training—is discussed. (For detailed discussion of the auditory training, see *Hearing Equals Behavior* by Guy Bérard.)

Cerebral Palsy

Finnie, Nancie R. 1975. *Handling the young cerebral palsied child at home.* New York: E. P. Dutton (337 pp.).

This is an indispensable guide for parents, nurses, therapists, doctors, and others caring for young children with cerebral palsy. The author includes a guide to community resources and suppliers of accessories and equipment as well as detailed suggestions for supplementing a treatment program by integrating training procedures. Especially helpful for new parents are sections on abnormal postures and movements and problems parents have with handling and daily care.

Geralis, Elaine. 1991. *Children with cerebral palsy: A parent's guide.* Rockville, Md.: Woodbine House (434 pp.).

This volume is essential reading for parents who want to learn about cerebral palsy and its impact on their child and family. Highly stressed is the importance of the family in assisting the child with cerebral palsy to lead a productive, satisfying life. *Children with Cerebral Palsy* includes contributions from doctors, therapists, educators, and parents, all of whom provide useful information and support. Information on many topics, including diagnosis, assessment, treatments, development, daily care, and legal rights, is provided. The authors also deal with grief, anger, and guilt in a compassionate and open manner. A glossary of important terms, reading list, and resource guide are included.

Hunt, Mimi, and Sally Weiss, eds. 1992. *Each of us remembers . . . . : Parents of children with cerebral palsy answer your questions.* Washington, D.C.: United Cerebral Palsy Association (32 pp.).

This booklet offers a chance for several parents to share with others what they have learned about having a child with cerebral palsy. Each parent answers questions that they wanted to ask when they received their children's diagnoses. Also included is a list of terms, with clear definitions, that are used in a diagnosis of cerebral palsy. The aim of this booklet is not only to answer questions but also to help new parents of children with cerebral palsy realize that they are not alone in the struggles they face.

Down's Syndrome

Pueschel, Siegfried M. 1990. *A parent's guide to Down's syndrome: Toward a brighter future.* Baltimore: Paul H. Brookes (315 pp.).

The author of this sensitive guide is the parent of a child with Down's syndrome. He has helped families around the world in coping with Down's syndrome. Pueschel discusses important developmental changes in the child and significant steps from infancy to adolescence. He provides simple explanations and advice on many pertinent topics. Sibling relationships, explanations to outsiders, educational considerations, and future quality of life are openly discussed with reassurance and strength. Referenced and suggested readings are also included.

Stray-Gundersen, Karen. 1986. *Babies with Down syndrome.* Rockville, Md.: Woodbine House (235 pp.).

> Written by professionals and parents, this book covers everything new parents need to know about raising babies with Down's syndrome in a loving environment. Up-to-date information on subjects important to the new parent, such as adjustment, daily care, and family life, is explored with sensitivity and thoroughness. Also provided is a section on early intervention and the teaching of a baby with Down's syndrome.

EPILEPSY

Reisner, Helen. 1988. *Children with epilepsy.* Rockville, Md.: Woodbine House (314 pp.).

> Vital current information and reassurance are offered in this volume to parents who face a long-misunderstood condition. The author gives a thorough explanation of epilepsy and discusses strategies for adjusting to this disorder. Important subjects such as development of high self-esteem in the epileptic child and the assessment of special needs are explored in a clear and compassionate style. A reading list, cassette list, and resource guide are also included.

GENERAL TOPICS

Anderson, Winifred; Stephan Chitwood; and Deidre Hayden. 1990. *Negotiating the special education maze: A guide for parents and teachers.* Rockville, Md.: Woodbine House (269 pp.).

> This well-organized, step-by-step guide is a valuable tool for anyone who works with the special education system or is involved in the education of a child with special needs. The guide discusses strategies for helping parents to be effective advocates for their children. Suggestions are also given for ways they can participate in educational decisions that concern them. Included is a wide range of current information on special education services and options, as well as checklists, exercises, and charts. Each step in the special education process is explained clearly and thoroughly. Appendixes include state and federal agencies and organizations dealing with specific disabilities.

Batshaw, Mark L., and Yvonne M. Perret. 1993. *Children with disabilities: A medical primer.* Baltimore: Paul H. Brookes (664 pp.).

> This universal resource book offers vital information on causes and effects of disabling conditions, characteristics of specific disabilities, and diagnostic and intervention strategies. Also explored are contemporary societal issues affecting children and families. Illustrations, charts, graphs, case studies, a glossary, and a section on syndromes are included.

Bérard, Guy. 1993. *Hearing equals behavior.* New Canaan, Conn.: Keats (178 pp.). In this book, Dr. Bérard explains the auditory training approach he developed. This approach has been helpful to people who have conditions such as hyperactivity, dyslexia, suicidal depression, and autism. He discusses the nature of the hearing process and several hearing disorders and their impact on behavior. He also explains how he developed and applied the auditory training approach, tells how to determine if an individual's behavior problems are caused by hearing problems, and discusses the apparatus used for testing and training. (See also *The Sound of a Miracle* by Annabel Stehli.)

Callanan, Charles R. 1990. *Since Owen: A parent to parent guide for the care of the disabled child.* Baltimore: Johns Hopkins University Press (466 pp.). Unique in its "family approach" to raising a child with disabilities, *Since Owen* gives parents information they need. It answers a wide range of specific questions and suggests further resources that can help parents become knowledgeable partners with their child's professionals. It explores topics ranging from genetic counseling to placement in an institution and causes of birth defects to raising a child with special needs. A concluding section looks at the disabled child as an adult and discusses topics such as living arrangements and religion. Most important, it gives families the message that they are not alone.

Des Jardins, Charlotte. 1993. *How to get services by being assertive.* Chicago: Family Resource Center on Disabilities (208 pp.). This book, written for parents of children with disabilities and the professionals who work with them, offers helpful advice for all caregivers who need or desire services for a care receiver. Readers of this book will learn the difference between assertive and nonassertive behaviors; ways to develop positive attitudes and eliminate negative ones; and how to use assertiveness in working with professionals, bureaucrats, and public officials. The author includes several success stories and information on available resources for parents and professionals.

Des Jardins, Charlotte. 1993. *How to organize an effective parent/advocacy group and move bureaucracies.* Chicago: Family Resource Center on Disabilities (270 pp.). Written for parents of children with disabilities and the professionals who work with them, this practical handbook is for any caregiver who wishes to become an advocate for caregivers and care receivers. The author offers helpful tips on how to set up parent/advocacy groups, effectively move bureaucracies to attain services, and teach children to become advocates for themselves by being positive and assertive. She also includes several success stories and helpful information on laws and legislation for parents, professionals, and children. A list of parent training and information centers and federal agencies is included.

Dickman, Irving R. 1993. *One miracle at a time: Getting help for a child with a disability.* Rev. ed. New York: Fireside (383 pp.).

This inspiring handbook offers the most recent information available on the new developments that are changing the future for disabled children, from saving at-risk newborns, to advances in assistive technology, to the pros and cons of full inclusion in education. This book not only provides practical advice and encouragement for parents of disabled children but also includes an extensive resource list of support organizations and associations.

Fitton, Pat. 1994. *Listen to me: Communicating the needs of people with profound intellectual and multiple disabilities.* Bristol, Pa.: Jessica Kingsley Publishers (244 pp.).

Listen to Me is a practical guide for parents and professionals coping with the complex problems of people with multiple disabilities. It offers information on asserting their rights, interpreting their needs successfully, and maintaining effective contact with professionals and organizations who deal with them. Pat Fitton uses examples from her own personal experiences with her disabled daughter to show how important it is to communicate that person's rights and needs in particular situations. She shows how it is possible to enrich the life of a person with profound disabilities and ensure that others value the person as an individual.

McAnaney, Kate Divine. 1992. *I wish: Dreams and realities of parenting a special needs child.* Sacramento: UCPA of California (87 pp.).

This is a book about conflict, courage, and creative solutions. McAnaney tells what it is like to be the parent of a disabled child and gives new perspective to professionals who work with exceptional families. In a conversational style, the author addresses guilt, grief, relaxation, and patience. Also included are messages from adults with disabilities who offer hope and inspiration.

McWilliam, P. J. 1993. *Working together with children and families.* Baltimore: Paul H. Brookes (310 pp.).

All the case studies in this book are based on actual experiences of professionals working in early intervention with families of children with disabilities. Written in a narrative format, the case studies are more comparable to short stories than academic readings. The characteristics of the children and families are diverse, as are the settings in which services are provided. This book offers clear pictures of children without labels, families with unique values, and professionals with feelings of their own.

Mills, Joyce C. 1992. *Little tree: A story for children with serious medical problems.* New York: Magination Press (32 pp.).

This sensitive story addresses the emotional difficulties of a child with a serious illness and offers a powerful healing metaphor that the child will remember after the book is closed. Medical procedures are subtly and symbolically mirrored with messages of hope and healing.

Rainforth, Beverly. 1992. *Collaborative teams for students with severe disabilities.* Baltimore: Paul H. Brookes (284 pp.).

Educational teams serving students with severe disabilities are entering an exciting and challenging era. Educational team members now have opportunities to play significant roles in helping children and youths with severe disabilities to achieve fulfilling, integrated lives. The authors of this book discuss the philosophical, legal, and programmatic foundations of collaborative teamwork, the process of designing individualized education programs, and implementation strategies and issues.

Seligman, Milton. 1989. *Ordinary families, special children.* New York: Guilford Press (272 pp.).

Families with children who have a disability are just like other families; however, the crisis of giving birth to a child with a disability thrusts family members into a situation that may make their lives different from those of other families. Discussions of this situation include social systems and family systems, becoming the parent of a disabled child, continuing adaptation, effects on family, models of intervention, cultural reactions, and professional-family interaction.

Simons, Robin. 1987. *After the tears: Parents talk about raising a child with a disability.* San Diego: Harcourt Brace Jovanovich (89 pp.).

In this book, Simons helps parents decide that they can continue to lead the lives they had planned—and incorporate their special-needs children into it. Included are stories of parents who have chosen this path, sharing their experiences and offering encouragement. Subjects such as guilt and anger, sorrow, personal growth, marital stress, and the future are explored with sensitivity.

Turnbull, Ann P.; Joan M. Patterson; Shirley K. Behr; Douglas L. Murphy; Janet G. Marquis; and Martha J. Blue-Banning. 1993. *Cognitive coping, families, and disability.* Baltimore: Paul H. Brookes (321 pp.).

Cognitive Coping, Families, and Disability provides insights into family adjustment and adaptation to stress, research findings on coping strategies, and determinants of individual coping and coping style. Through a participatory research process, the authors gained valuable information on empirical, theoretical, clinical, and consumer perspectives about disability and cognitive coping. The book presents this information and provides professionals with a clear-cut research agenda.

Turnbull, Ann P., and H. Rutherford Turnbull III. 1990. *Families, professionals, and exceptionality: A special partnership.* 2d ed. New York: Merrill (485 pp.).

Families, Professionals, and Exceptionality: A Special Partnership concerns families, people who have disabilities, professionals, and ways they can work together more effectively. This book helps current and future professionals understand the diversity in families, family interaction, and family functions.

Strategies for better communication between families and professionals are explored as well as ways to help families better cope with their situations. Professional ethics and morals are discussed, as well as when and if the use of the law is warranted. An extensive appendix with lists of resources for families and professionals is included.

Mental Retardation

Smith, Romayne. 1993. *Children with mental retardation: A parent's guide.* Rockville, Md.: Woodbine House (437 pp.).

> This comprehensive guide covers mild to moderate retardation that has been diagnosed at birth or in early childhood. The authors discuss the emotional impact of the diagnosis on parents, as well as the challenges such a diagnosis presents. Thoroughly explored are subjects of development, evaluation, special education, and daily living of the mentally retarded child. Valuable strategies for coping and acceptance are presented for parents. Experiences of other families are expressed through parent statements to offer insight and reassurance to new parents of children with mental retardation.

Trainer, Marilyn. 1991. *Differences in common: Straight talk on mental retardation, Down syndrome, and life.* Rockville, Md.: Woodbine House (231 pp.).

> A collection of almost fifty essays, *Differences in Common* speaks not only to a parent of a child that is "different" but also to those who know little about people with mental retardation. Trainer brings a fresh, candid outlook to the challenges, hopes, and fears of family life—a life shaped by a child with Down's syndrome, but one that strikes a common chord in all of us.

CHRONIC ILLNESS

Biegel, David E.; Esther Sales; and Richard Schulz. 1991. *Family caregiving in chronic illness.* Newbury Park, Calif.: Sage (331 pp.).

> This volume provides a comprehensive analysis of the role and function of family caregiving within and across adult populations with dependency needs because of chronic disease. Five specific diseases are examined: cancer, heart disease, stroke, Alzheimer's disease, and mental illness. The authors provide a synthesis of existing research knowledge about family caregiving of dependent adult populations and suggest new directions for research and practice. Trends leading to the emergence of caregiving are carefully examined as a major societal issue. Intervention models are examined, as well as research findings pertaining to the effectiveness of particular interventions.

Funk, Sandra G. 1993. *Key aspects of caring for the chronically ill.* New York: Springer (350 pp.).

This comprehensive sourcebook contains information on many aspects of caring for the chronically ill. In the overview, the author includes discussions of hospitalized chronically ill, transitions from hospital to home, home care, living with chronic illness, and research findings regarding the chronically ill. There is a special section covering issues concerning chronically ill children.

Goldfarb, Lori A.; Mary Jane Brotherson; Jean Ann Summers; and Ann P. Turnbull. 1986. *Meeting the challenge of disability or chronic illness: A family guide.* Baltimore: Paul H. Brookes (181 pp.).

This practical tool for family problem solving can help ease the pain of difficult times and turn disappointments into triumphs. Part 1, "Taking Stock," will help families dealing with disability or chronic illness take an "inventory" of their family, identify their values and the resources available to them, and further strengthen those resources. Part 2, "Problem Solving," is a carefully thought-out process based on simplicity. The step-by-step method will help families to find solutions more quickly to the issues they face.

Lyons, Renee F.; Michael J. L. Sullivan; and Paul G. Ritvo. 1995. *Relationships in chronic illness and disability.* Thousand Oaks, Calif.: Sage (189 pp.).

This book deals with the interpersonal issues that arise when relationships evolve under the challenges of chronic illness. Three interactive relationship-illness processes are examined: relationship change, supports and stressors, and relationship-focused coping. Intervention in close relationships to improve coping with illness is also discussed.

Maurer, Janet R. 1989. *Building a new dream.* New York: Addison-Wesley (307 pp.).

Building a New Dream is a compassionate and practical guide to understanding and coping with the emotional and social aspects of chronic illness and disability. The author explains how to work with health professionals to learn about one's illness and find resources, how to come to terms with emotional strain in order to cope with depression, and how to cope with the changing roles that illness brings about for all involved.

Pitzele, Sefra K. 1985. *We are not alone: Learning to live with chronic illness.* New York: Workman (315 pp.).

We Are Not Alone offers inspiration and practical living strategies to millions of Americans suffering from chronic illnesses and priceless advice for those who care for them. Drawing on firsthand experiences, the author is a friendly guide to coping with every aspect of chronic impairment, from overcoming the trauma of the diagnosis to managing daily routines with humor, dignity, and hope.

Pollin, Irene, and Susan K. Golant. 1994. *Taking charge: Overcoming the challenges of long-term illness.* New York: Random House (255 pp.).

In *Taking Charge*, the authors explain the method of medical crisis counseling, which Pollin pioneered to help people survive the crisis of long-term illness and live productively. Eight common fears (such as fear of loss of control, fear of abandonment, and fear of death) of those dealing with long-term illness are identified, and strategies are provided to help overcome them.

Register, Cheri. 1987. *Living with chronic illness: Days of patience and passion*. New York: Free Press (316 pp.).

> *Living with Chronic Illness* explores the shifting emotions involved in dealing with chronic illness, including the confusion and uncertainty that precede diagnosis and the unexpected relief that often comes when the nature of the illness is finally confirmed. Register illuminates patience as a way of life and discusses how it feels to know that disease will always be there. She also acknowledges that anger, fear, and grief can be appropriate, healthy responses to physical suffering.

Strong, Maggie. 1988. *Mainstay: For the well spouse of the chronically ill*. New York: Penguin Books (329 pp.).

> *Mainstay* is a book about living with a chronically ill spouse. Maggie Strong tells her own story and shows that living with someone who is chronically ill is more than just hard work. She raised her family, managed her house and family finances, maintained her career, and safeguarded her own emotional and physical needs while caring for her husband, who has multiple sclerosis. Strong writes of the emotional toll experienced, from keeping anger and guilt tucked away to being constantly aware that the situation will only get worse. The chapters are full of concrete, vital information on how to cope with the challenges of long-term illnesses. *Mainstay* is a book that will inspire courage and strength in all those who live with people who are chronically ill.

Walsh, Froma, and Carol M. Anderson, eds. 1988. *Chronic disorders and the family*. New York: Haworth Press (183 pp.).

> The authors examine the role of the family in understanding and treating severe and chronic mental and physical illnesses. The goal is to increase awareness of the problems facing families coping with severe disorders. Topics such as schizophrenia, depression, anxiety disorders, eating disorders, and substance abuse are thoroughly explored, including research findings and therapy strategies.

CONGREGATIONAL CAREGIVING

Building Community Supports Project. 1994. *Dimensions of faith and congregational ministries with persons with developmental disabilities and their families*. Piscataway, N.J.: University Affiliated Program of New Jersey (56 pp.).

> This guide includes a bibliography and a list of addresses of resources for clergy, laypersons, families, and service providers. These resources are divided by areas of interest and program/ministry. Examples of topics and information

included are worship and sacraments, theological issues, parents and families of persons with disabilities, youth groups and adult education, pastoral counseling, and reading and audio/visual resources.

Harbaugh, Gary L. 1992. *Caring for the caregiver: Growth models for professional leaders and congregations.* Washington, D.C.: Alban Institute (117 pp.).

This book is especially aimed at the clergy, reminding them of their responsibility to care for themselves as well as for others. It challenges congregations and churches to provide preventive care and ongoing support as well as crisis intervention. Helpful information at the end of the book includes a "caring for the caregiver" survey and a listing of resources.

Ransom, Judy G. 1994. *The courage to care: Seven families touched by disability and congregational caring.* Nashville: Upper Room Books (205 pp.).

This book is a collection of stories about seven different families who are struggling with different disabilities and finding help through congregational caring. Each story is unique and moving, but all demonstrate the impact of caring congregations during times of difficulty. Appendixes include guidelines for helping and a listing of resources and organizations.

COPING AND SELF-CARE FOR THE CAREGIVER

Carter, Rosalynn. 1994. *Helping yourself help others: A book for caregivers.* New York: Times Books (278 pp.).

Helping Yourself Help Others was written to inform, encourage, empathize with, and advocate for informal (family and lay) caregivers. It also provides valuable insights for professional caregivers. Rosalynn Carter discusses the feelings of caregivers; provides information about what caring means; explains the stages of caregiving; and offers ideas, information, and advice to people currently providing care and to future caregivers. This guidebook offers practical solutions to caregivers' typical problems. It was written with empathy and sensitivity to help caregivers meet a difficult challenge head-on and find fulfillment and empowerment in their caregiving roles. More than fifty pages are devoted to addresses and phone numbers of organizations and a list of books helpful to caregivers.

Cole, Harry A. 1991. *Helpmates: Support in times of critical illness.* Louisville, Ky.: Westminster/John Knox Press (157 pp.).

In this book, written by a caregiving spouse for other caregivers, author Harry Cole recognizes that caregivers who provide help for dependent loved ones are often unprepared to cope with the physical and emotional effects that accompany long-term illness. Making use of interviews with many people involved in caring for loved ones who are critically or terminally ill, Cole gives direction and support to help caregivers gain more patience and understanding.

Collins, Sheila K. 1992. *Stillpoint: The dance of self-caring, self-healing.* Fort Worth, Tex.: TLC Productions (201 pp.).

> *Stillpoint* is a practical self-help book for anyone who is a caregiver at work and/or in family life. The author states that people who care for others often have trouble caring for themselves (physically, mentally, emotionally, and spiritually) and that failure to care for oneself may lead to loss of ability to care for others. The book will help readers increase their understanding of themselves; identify the missing elements in their self-caring lifestyles; learn how to alter their environments to support self-care; and learn self-caring skills to take care of themselves while caring for others.

Dempcy, Mary, and Rene Tihista. 1991. *Stress personalities: A look inside ourselves.* Bolinas, Calif.: Focal Point Press (233 pp.).

> This book discusses seven types of stress personalities many people possess and their effects on relationships and health. The book helps readers identify their own stress personalities and learn how these affect their lives. At the end of each section, the authors offer new, positive behaviors to practice in order to counteract the respective stress personality behaviors that are unproductive and detrimental.

Hover, Margot. 1994. *Caring for yourself when caring for others.* Mystic, Conn.: Twenty-third Publications (74 pp.).

> The author uses Scripture, personal stories, situational experiences, and prayer to offer practical and uplifting support for caregivers. She offers simple, direct advice for dealing with everyday occurrences facing those who give care to others. She also offers ways that caregivers can nourish themselves and revitalize their efforts.

Karr, Katherine L. 1992. *Taking time for me: How caregivers can effectively deal with stress.* Buffalo, N.Y.: Prometheus Books (175 pp.).

> Family caregivers must often juggle their duties as parents, spouses, and employees while tending to the daily needs of a loved one who is elderly, chronically ill, or dying. For these people, stress often becomes an everyday occurrence that at times seems insurmountable. Karr's insightful observations and suggestions—enhanced by personal accounts of real care providers who are struggling with their own needs while tending to the needs of others—demonstrate that caregivers can overcome their personal conflicts and develop innovative ways of renewing their strength without jeopardizing the well-being of those who depend on them.

Kleinke, Chris L. 1990. *Coping with life challenges.* Pacific Grove, Calif.: Brooks/Cole (240 pp.).

> This easy-to-understand guide helps the reader learn to cope with illness, pain, loss, anger, failure, and conflict. Whether the difficulties are minor or serious, presented in this book are coping strategies that can help anyone regain a sense

of control in his or her life. The author presents a "how-to" approach and practical suggestions for making the information work for the reader.

Schlossberg, Nancy K. 1994. *Overwhelmed: Coping with life's ups and downs.* New York: Lexington Books (154 pp.).

All of us face transitions or turning points in our lives. How we handle these journeys, live through them, and learn from them is what this book is about. The author discusses the transition process, how to take stock of one's situation and oneself, and how to take charge of the changes in one's life. Her prescription for coping is mature, sympathetic, and realistic.

Sherman, James R. 1994. *Creative caregiving.* Golden Valley, Minn.: Pathway Books (84 pp.).

This book helps caregivers develop creative ways to relieve the difficult aspects of their caregiving. The author discusses creativity and caregiving, barriers to creative caregiving, the seven components needed for creativity, and how to develop one's creative talents. Checklists and exercises help the reader become a more creative caregiver.

Sherman, James R. 1994. *Positive caregiver attitudes.* Golden Valley, Minn.: Pathway Books (84 pp.).

This is an important manual for any caregiver. It is loaded with down-to-earth strategies for developing and maintaining positive attitudes toward care receivers, caregiving, and life in general. This book also identifies the sources of negative feelings and illustrates their destructive effects. It is filled with simple rules, commonsense ideas, and self-help exercises.

Sherman, James R. 1994. *Preventing caregiver burnout.* Golden Valley, Minn.: Pathway Books (76 pp.).

Caregivers work long hours under constant emotional pressure and can lose their motivation and commitment to caregiving. This book addresses this fact. It describes what burnout is, what causes it, and the effects it has on the burned-out person. Lastly, the author presents easy-to-follow procedures for preventing burnout and maintaining an optimistic outlook toward caregiving. Checklists and self-help exercises are included.

Sherman, James R. 1995. *The magic of humor in caregiving.* Golden Valley, Minn.: Pathway Books (93 pp.).

This book explains the well-established healing benefits of laughter and humor in reducing stress. It shows how playfulness and humor can be used to increase personal effectiveness, promote wellness, and lighten the impact of one's caregiving. Self-rating checklists and self-help exercises help readers evaluate the extent to which humor is currently a part of their lives and helps them learn how to increase the laughter in their lives.

Spencer, Sabina A., and John D. Adams. 1990. *Life changes: Growing through personal transitions.* San Luis Obispo, Calif.: Impact (192 pp.).

Helping readers cope with the inevitable personal transitions in life is the focus of this book. Caregivers can use *Life Changes* as a tool to give them suggestions for coping with their caregiving demands. The contents include life changes, the seven stages of transition, where to find support, developing and utilizing skills to deal with change, keeping a positive attitude, staying healthy, managing stress, and living with change.

DIABETES

Krall, Leo P. 1989. *Joslin diabetes manual.* Malvern, Pa.: Lea & Febiges (406 pp.).
This instructional guide is full of detailed information concerning people with diabetes. Its aim is to assist diabetics to understand the disorder and to learn how to live full and healthy lives. The author thoroughly describes the process of diabetes, the different types, and their causes and symptoms. The issues of nutrition, exercise, treatments, and pregnancy are also covered in the chapters.

Schafer, Walt. 1992. *Stress management for wellness.* 2d ed. Orlando, Fla.: Harcourt (533 pp.).
This book will prove helpful for every person but especially to caregivers who are experiencing significant stress in their lives. It promotes an integrated, whole-person, lifestyle approach to stress management. Its goal is to assist readers to control and channel stress rather than succumb to it. Aspects of stress and coping included in this book are understanding stress and wellness, stress-related symptoms and disorders, Type A behavior and hostility, and methods of managing stress. Special applications applying to college stress and job stress are also included. Many tables, self-rating scales, and self-help exercises help readers analyze their own stress and coping behaviors.

EATING DISORDERS

Brownell, Kelly D., and John P. Foreyt, eds. 1986. *Handbook of eating disorders: Physiology, psychology, and treatment of obesity, anorexia, and bulimia.* New York: Basic Books (529 pp.).
This book is an important resource for professionals who work with people who have eating disorders—anorexia, bulimia, and obesity. Written by authorities in the field, it focuses on all aspects of these disorders—health consequences, epidemiology, inpatient and outpatient treatment.

Siegel, Michele; Judith Brisman; and Margot Weinshel. 1988. *Surviving an eating disorder: Strategies for family and friends.* New York: Harper & Row (222 pp.).
This book offers specific guidelines to help family and friends of people who have eating disorders. The authors offer rules and new behaviors/actions that

will encourage the recovery process. Psychological components of eating disorders and possible treatments are discussed. Other helpful books and organizations are included. Topics of this book include the behavioral, psychological, and family context of eating disorders; bringing the disorder out in the open; coping with denial; seeking help; disengaging from the eating disorder; and relating to the person, not the disorder.

ELDERLY AS CAREGIVERS

Minkler, Meredith. 1993. *Grandmothers as caregivers.* Newbury Park, Calif.: Sage (238 pp.).

This book contains discussions exploring the concerns of grandmothers as caregivers. The author looks at the health status of grandmother caregivers, economic considerations, support networks and social support, combining work and child care, raising children of the crack cocaine epidemic, and community interventions to support grandparent caregivers.

Roberto, Karen A., ed. 1993. *The elderly caregiver: Caring for adults with developmental disabilities.* Newbury Park, Calif.: Sage (216 pp.).

Roberto addresses the predominant issues and concerns confronting elder caregivers. She provides insight into the physical, psychological, and social needs of this growing segment of the population. The needs of elderly people caring for adult children, aging adults, and persons with specific disabilities are explored, including the increasing burden of caregiving, the ordeal of facing their own future, and planning for out-of-home placement. Case management is also examined.

GENERAL TOPICS

Bass, Deborah S. 1990. *Caring families: Supports and interventions.* Washington, D.C.: National Association of Social Workers (279 pp.).

In this volume, Bass provides a useful framework for understanding and assisting those who care for family members—both young and old. This book provides useful practice tools for assessing the strengths and needs of caregiving families and for assisting them in problem solving and in coping with the stresses of caregiving. *Caring Families* will be important to many audiences, helping professionals, public and private policy makers, and caregiving families. Addresses and phone numbers of state agencies responsible for health care, aging, maternal and child health, developmental disabilities, special education; VA medical centers and clinics; and Department of Defense family support programs are included.

Bernstein, Gail S., and Judith A. Halaszyn. 1989. *Human services? . . . That must be so rewarding: A practical guide for professional development.* Baltimore: Paul H. Brookes (171 pp.).

This easy-to-use resource contains practical insights and personal guidance for those involved in human services. Included are guidelines and suggestions for addressing personal motives, goals, and limits; discovering fundamental values for human services; developing effective work relationships; and identifying long-term professional goals. The author includes exercises throughout each chapter to assist readers in assessing themselves in a number of areas.

Boise, Linda, ed. N.d. *Helping families help themselves: Reaching the employed caregiver.* Portland, Oreg.: Family Support Services, Good Samaritan Hospital and Medical Center (15 pp.).

This booklet is for people and organizations that provide support or are considering developing programs for employed caregivers or who would like to know more about the special needs of working caregivers. It identifies their needs, offers information about programs and services that can help them, and offers advice on ways to reach them through the workplace and community programs. Topics include a profile of the employed caregiver, the challenges of working and caregiving, what employed caregivers need, benefits to business, how a survey can assess need, how focus groups help, ways to reach employed caregivers, offering programs in the workplace, and sample telephone scripts, letters, questions, and evaluation forms.

Caplan, Paula J. 1994. *You're smarter than they make you feel: How the experts intimidate us and what we can do about it.* New York: Free Press (212 pp.).

Drawing on a wealth of anecdotes along with current psychological research, Paula Caplan persuasively shows us that we do not need to feel stupid or powerless when dealing with experts in any field. She points out the techniques experts typically use to intimidate clients, why they employ these techniques, and why we blame ourselves. Caplan concludes by showing us how we can recognize the techniques of disempowerment, employ helpful counterstrategies, and think more critically in order to elicit the needed information or action.

Cicirelli, Victor G. 1992. *Family caregiving: Autonomous and paternalistic decision making.* Newbury Park, Calif.: Sage (252 pp.).

Family Caregiving offers researchers, practitioners, and professionals an informative look at a new area of inquiry—paternalism and respect for autonomy in family caregiving decision making. It clearly discusses family caregiving in long-term home care, the meaning of autonomy and paternalism, and the nature of dyadic family decision making. This volume emphasizes autonomy in family care as opposed to formal care and how lack of education, negative attitudes toward elders, and family traditions can influence the frequency of paternalistic decision making.

Committee on Handicaps. 1993. *Caring for people with physical impairment: The journey back.* Washington, D.C.: American Psychiatric Press (178 pp.).

This book brings together the expertise of caregivers from a variety of backgrounds to examine the special needs of patients with physical impairments. It explores clinical and educational applications to the caregiving of the physically impaired. Offered in this volume is information on coping strategies for the caregiver and on the special issues related to the rehabilitation process. The information will be helpful to both informal and formal caregivers.

Dixon, Barbara. 1994. *Good health for African Americans.* New York: Crown Publishers (414 pp.).

Good Health for African Americans defines the complex issues that account for the health gap between black and white Americans at all income levels and presents a self-help program for improving health. Dixon's message is clear and simple: By adopting a healthy diet and making lifestyle changes, African Americans can increase their chances for longer and more robust lives.

Doka, K. J. 1993. *Living with life-threatening illness: A guide for patients, their families, and caregivers.* New York: Lexington Books (261 pp.).

Provided in this book is a positive plan for improving the lives of seriously ill patients, their families, and caregivers. *Living with Life-Threatening Illness* gives us a new way of looking at the different stages of illness. The experience of living with illness is emphasized, rather than just anticipating its terminal phase. This book is essential for all who are dealing with major illness, whether personally or professionally.

Feetham, Suzanne L.; Susan B. Meister; Janice M. Bell; and Catherine L. Gilliss, eds. 1993. *The nursing of families: Theory/research/education/practice.* Newbury Park, Calif.: Sage (308 pp.).

The Nursing of Families offers significant directions for crosscutting issues in practice, education, research, and theory to help bridge the gap between perceived needs and expectations of families and the actual practice of nursing. Among the issues explored are policy and economic issues, theory development, research methodology, cross-cultural concerns, HIV/AIDS, and homeless mothers and children.

Gaut, Delores A. 1992. *The presence of caring in nursing.* Hudson Street, N.Y.: National League for Nursing Press (267 pp.).

This book is a collection of essays dealing with the topic of caring in nursing. Explored are the concepts of presence, spiritual connection, caring nursing environments, impact of nurses' caring on patients, conflict between caring and professionalization, and the magic of caring.

Gething, Lindsay. 1992. *Person to person: A guide for professionals working with people with disabilities.* Baltimore: Paul H. Brookes (267 pp.).

Gething looks at a great many aspects of different types of disabilities: physiology; treatment; social and emotional aspects; family reactions; education; employment; attitudes of others; and much more. Written with personal accounts, this guide is easy to read and sympathetic. It would be useful for the professional or the layperson who would like to learn more about the different aspects of impairment.

Grasha, Anthony F. 1995. *Practical applications of psychology.* 4th ed. New York: HarperCollins (476 pp.).

This book explores how psychology may be applied to the individual in everyday life. Readers are shown how to develop action plans to help them make more effective decisions, modify their behavior, communicate and relate to others better, manage stress, and develop positive self-images. Family caregivers would also find this text helpful.

Hayslip, Bert. 1992. *Hospice care.* Newbury Park, Calif.: Sage (235 pp.).

The intent of this volume is to serve as an introduction to hospice for new personnel, students, and volunteers. Its focus is toward the nonmedical aspects of patient care. Addressed are the issues of communication and assessment skills in hospice, special education role of hospice, working with the patient, working with families, and grief and bereavement.

Heath, Angela. 1993. *Long distance caregiving: A survival guide for far away caregivers.* Lakewood, Colo.: American Source Books (122 pp.).

Long Distance Caregiving is a helpful guide that provides step-by-step, practical suggestions for caregivers, especially caregivers who live some distance from their care receivers. Some of the topics included are travel tips, paperwork, legal and financial issues, adjusting one's care plan, and relocation. Checklists of suggestions, tips, and considerations and what should be done within specific time frames help organize caregivers. A list of helpful organizations appears at the end.

Hooyman, Nancy R., and Judith Gonyea. 1995. *Feminist perspectives on family care: Policies for gender justice.* Thousand Oaks, Calif.: Sage (418 pp.).

In *Feminist Perspectives on Family Care,* the authors examine caregiving as a feminist issue, looking at its impact on women socially, personally, and economically. They review how changing family structures, the changing economy and workforce, and the changing health care demands of needy adults have affected women's lives. They also critique existing public and private policies and the changes in social institutions and attitudes meant to improve the lives of women.

Horowitz, Karen E., and Douglas M. Lanes. 1992. *Witness to illness: Strategies for caregiving and coping.* Reading, Mass.: Addison-Wesley (277 pp.).

Witness to Illness speaks to our feelings of helplessness, and perhaps hopelessness, when we are unable to do anything to restore health to a loved one.

Horowitz and Lanes show us that we do not have to be passive. This book follows the course of events in a typical illness—from handling the initial bad news, through caregiving, to the long-term effects of the illness—and suggests specific, practical ways in which we can actively contribute to the survival and well-being of people we care for and about.

Kahana, Eva; David E. Biegel; and May L. Wykle. 1994. *Family caregiving across the lifespan.* Thousand Oaks, Calif.: Sage (418 pp.).

Family Caregiving across the Lifespan considers the broad spectrum of chronic illnesses that require family caregiving throughout the life span and includes in its focus both members of the family caregiving relationship and significant nonfamily caregivers. The authors also explore the social context in which care is provided, devoting an entire section to discussions of interaction between informal and formal caregivers and society at large. The value of providing support to caregivers, including caregivers of persons with AIDS, is discussed.

Larson, Dale G. 1993. *The helper's journey: Working with people facing grief, loss, and life-threatening illness.* Champaign, Ill.: Research Press (279 pp.).

This book is for caregivers—professional and family. It is divided into three main sections. Part 1 focuses on the personal experiences of helping, such as emotional involvement and handling stress. Part 2 discusses the interpersonal dimensions of caregiving, focusing on helping relationships and communication skills. Part 3 deals with helping teams and support groups and how they can benefit healing.

Lassiter, Sybil M. 1995. *Multicultural clients: A professional handbook for health care providers and social workers.* Westport, Conn.: Greenwood Press (194 pp.).

This text provides basic information to health care providers who work with multicultural clients. The author presents the following cultural groups: African, Arab, Chinese, Cuban, East Indian, Filipino, German, Haitian, Irish, Italian, Japanese, Jewish, Korean, Mexican, and Vietnamese Americans and discusses their population numbers, economic status, major illnesses, and death rates in the United States. Lassiter makes comparisons of orientations toward family, the elderly, child rearing, socialization, health beliefs and practices, dietary patterns, religious beliefs and practices, and beliefs about death and dying for each cultural group.

Lechner, Viola M., and Michael A. Creedon. 1994. *Managing work and family life.* New York: Springer (187 pp.).

In this addition to the professional literature on the changing needs of families and working caregivers, the authors identify and discuss emerging family-sensitive corporate- and government-sponsored programs and employee benefits. They describe the full range of workplace responses and focus on policies (for example, the Family Medical Leave Act of 1993) and programs (such as flextime, job sharing, and compressed workweeks). Lechner and Creedon delineate a seven-step program-development model for labor unions and companies interested in planning and implementing family-focused workplace programs.

Locke, Don C. 1992. *Increasing multicultural understanding: A comprehensive model.* Newbury Park, Calif.: Sage (166 pp.).

This book sets forth the process necessary to implement effective education and counseling strategies for culturally diverse populations. It is designed to provide one of the necessary steps in accomplishing the task of gaining an overview of various cultural groups. It will help the reader identify characteristics of cultures, make comparisons between the dominant culture and culturally different groups, and use that information to develop strategies or interventions for students or clients. Readers will become more aware of their own ethnocentrism and increase their awareness of the role culture plays in determining the ways people think, feel, and act.

Lowe, Paula C. 1993. *Carepooling: How to get the help you need to care for the ones you love.* San Francisco: Berrett-Koehler Publishers (292 pp.).

Carepooling offers simple, practical ways to exchange help and share support with friends, neighbors, and co-workers. Enlivened by stories of more than two hundred caregivers, this book provides the tools to identify potential carepoolers, understand why it is hard to ask for help, initiate carepooling relationships, resolve conflicts among carepoolers, and hire a shared care provider.

Lustbader, Wendy. 1991. *Counting on kindness: The dilemmas of dependency.* New York: Free Press (206 pp.).

Vividly illustrated with true stories and quotations and full of insights from Wendy Lustbader's clinical experience, *Counting on Kindness* explores issues of power and dependency and shows how to regain a sense of power and purpose while dependent on others. She discusses such issues as coping with too much time on one's hands, learning to think of the past productively, handling regret and feelings of uselessness, and reviving one's self-esteem in the face of debility.

MacNamara, Roger Dale. 1992. *Creating abuse-free caregiving environments for children, the disabled, and the elderly: Preparing, supervising, and managing caregivers for the emotional impact of their responsibilities.* Springfield, Ill.: Charles C. Thomas (256 pp.).

MacNamara takes the position that professional caregivers must be able, stable, and self-renewing to avoid becoming abusive. In this manual, the author explores the topic of abuse and its relationship to environment and stress and describes a series of abuser "profiles." He also offers strategies for avoiding or stopping abusive behaviors.

Maguire, Lambert. 1991. *Social support systems in practice: A generalist approach.* Silver Spring, Md.: National Association of Social Workers Press (177 pp.).

This book for social work practitioners is designed to be a practical guide to using social support systems. The author examines the variety of ways in which social work practitioners can organize family, friends, and fellow professionals into therapeutic, rehabilitative, or preventive units of help for clients. The book describes three different approaches to such social support systems but maintains a generalist orientation.

Mayeroff, Milton. 1971. *On caring.* Scranton, Pa.: HarperCollins (123 pp.).

A generalized description of caring and an account of how caring can give comprehensive meaning and order to one's life are the themes dealt with in this book. It is a short, beautifully written account of what it means to live a full, happy, and connected life and how to help others come to do this. Mayeroff makes the reader aware of what caring involves in a clear and engaging style.

McDaniel, Susan H.; Jeri Hepworth; and William J. Doherty. 1992. *Medical family therapy: A biopsychosocial approach to families with health problems.* New York: Basic Books (295 pp.).

In *Medical Family Therapy,* the authors detail their medical family therapy model, a biopsychosocial family systems approach that operates in collaboration with patients, families, health care professionals, and community groups. The goal is to coordinate care for the benefit of people who are ill and their families/caregivers.

Miller, James E. 1995. *When you're the caregiver: Twelve things to do if someone you care for is ill or incapacitated. When you're ill or incapacitated: Twelve things to remember in times of sickness, injury, or disability.* Ft. Wayne, Ind.: Willowgreen (62 pp.).

This book is written for the caregiver *and* the care receiver. The author combines his knowledge as an ordained clergyman and grief counselor to offer words of spiritual comfort and advice to help facilitate a cooperative, working partnership between the caregiver and care receiver and to increase each partner's ability to cope with the situation.

Nisbet, Jan. 1992. *Natural supports in school, at work, and in the community for people with severe disabilities.* Baltimore: Paul H. Brookes (362 pp.).

Promoting the position that assistance must be defined by the needs of individuals rather than the requirements of service "systems," this definitive book combines thoughtful research and provocative first-person accounts to give fresh insight and practical guidance for using natural supports. Thoughtful chapters supply essential information on strategies for building community membership for individuals with disabilities, on support programs and networks available, on the role of natural supports in public schools, and much more.

Nottingham, Jack, and Joanne Nottingham, eds. 1990. *The professional and family caregiver: Dilemmas, rewards, and new directions.* Americus, Ga.: Rosalynn

Carter Institute for Human Development, Georgia Southwestern State University (77 pp.).

The presentations given at the inaugural conference of the Rosalynn Carter Institute for Human Development in 1990 at Georgia Southwestern State University in Americus, Georgia, are contained in this book. Topics include caregiving in the United States, shared responsibility, caring for the caregiver, caregiving in a holistic context, senior citizen caregivers, caring for the chronically and mentally ill, professional and family caregiving from medical and social work perspectives, health and mental health care in the future, and the caring community.

Pugach, Marleen C., and Lawrence J. Johnson. 1995. *Collaborative practitioners/ collaborative schools.* Denver: Love Publishing (265 pp.).

This book stresses collaboration among professionals, families, and students in schools. However, many of the principles are applicable to health care, its providers, caregiving families, and care receivers. The emphasis is on teamwork to enhance services and benefit the people involved. Topics include collaboration (what it is, how to do it, and participation); communication (skills to facilitate, and barriers to, effective communication); and collaboration (working with and supporting groups, and school-university and school-family collaboration).

Rolland, John S. 1994. *Families, illness, and disability: An integrative treatment model.* New York: Basic Books (309 pp.).

Using his Family Systems Illness Model, the author shows how the biopsychosocial demands of different illnesses and disabilities create particular strains on the family, how the stages of an illness affect the family, how family legacies of loss and illness shape their coping responses, and how family belief systems play a crucial role in the ability to manage health and illness. Practitioners will learn how to help families live well despite physical limitations and the uncertainties of threatened loss; encourage empowering rather than shame-based illness narratives; rewrite rigid caregiving scripts; and encourage intimacy and maximize autonomy for all family members. This is an ideal book for all health and mental health professionals and students who work with illness, disability, and loss in a wide variety of clinical settings.

Roter, Debra L., and Judith A. Hall. 1993. *Doctors talking with patients/patients talking with doctors: Improving communication in medical visits.* Westport, Conn.: Auburn House (203 pp.).

Medical visits are not as effective and satisfying as they would be if doctors and patients communicated better with each other. Roter and Hall set out specific, scientifically established principles and recommendations for improving doctor-patient relationships. Improved communication will aid understanding, improve motivation, encourage the pursuit of medical advice, and reduce negative psychological/emotional reactions, especially for patients.

Salisbury, Christine L., and James Intagliata. 1986. *Respite care: Support for persons with developmental disabilities and their families.* Baltimore: Paul H. Brookes (315 pp.).

This book is about providing respite care for families who have a member with a disability. *Respite Care* represents an effort to respond to the growing need for information on respite care and family support services by providing readers with a perspective on the rationale for and design and evaluation of respite care programs. The chapters provide a wealth of practical information presented against a background of theory and research supporting the need for respite services. The reader will gain an understanding of the issues surrounding the establishment of respite programs.

Sawa, Russell J., ed. 1992. *Family health care.* Newbury Park, Calif.: Sage (297 pp.). This collection presents an assortment of ways of talking about families, analyzing their effects on health and illness, and assessing the family coping strategies and how effective they are. In doing this, the author relates family pathology and therapy to concerns of primary care. Sections cover family theories and primary health care, research on family health care, and education and practice of professionals dealing with families.

Schaufeli, Wilmar B.; Christina Maslach; and Tadeusz Marek, eds. 1993. *Professional burnout: Recent developments in theory and research.* Washington, D.C.: Taylor & Francis (292 pp.).

A rapidly growing number of people experience psychological strain at their workplaces. Results of this include higher rates of absenteeism and turnover and an increasing number of workers receiving disability benefits because of psychological problems. This book focuses on one specific kind of occupational stress: burnout, the depletion of energy resources as a result of continuous emotional demands of the job. There are five sections to the book: interpersonal approaches, individual approaches, organizational approaches, methodological issues, and the future outlook of burnout.

Shields, Craig V. 1987. *Strategies: A practical guide for dealing with professionals and human service systems.* Richmond Hill, Ontario: Human Services Press (144 pp.). This handbook answers many common questions, discusses situations and problems typically faced when dealing with human service providers, and offers strategies for dealing with them. Shields helps the reader understand professionals and become familiar with the "system." Considerations for selecting a professional or agency and dealing with personnel are explored in detail. A particularly helpful master list of strategies is included in the appendix.

Singer, George H. S., and Larry K. Irvin, eds. 1989. *Support for caregiving families:*

Enabling positive adaptation to disability. Baltimore: Paul H. Brookes (348 pp.).

> These authors present an overview of family support services for families of individuals with developmental disabilities. The services described in the book aim to create productive partnerships between social services and families in order to help families succeed in their caregiving roles without supplanting them. Content is organized around the roles of family stress and the concept of the family life cycle.

Singer, George H. S.; Laurie E. Powers; and Ardis L. Olson. 1996. *Redefining family support: Innovations in public-private partnerships.* Baltimore: Paul H. Brookes (477 pp.).

> This resource examines family support practices, policies, and strategies. It outlines various programs and funding options for meeting the diverse needs of families who care for a family member who has a disability. Topics include family support for families of people with special needs, family support across populations, and issues and innovations in public policy.

Stevenson, Robert G., ed. 1994. *What will we do?: Preparing a school community to cope with crises.* Amityville, N.Y.: Baywood Publishing (214 pp.).

> *What Will We Do?* was written to train school personnel to help victims cope with crises. Although this book is aimed at schools, health care and other professionals could benefit from the information, resources, and techniques discussed. Topics include preparing schools for crisis management; crises of youth suicide, HIV/AIDS, and violence; support groups and the role of peer support; and critical incident stress debriefing.

Unger, Donald G., and Douglas R. Powell, eds. 1991. *Families as nurturing systems: Support across the life span.* Binghamton, N.Y.: Haworth (251 pp.).

> In this volume, Unger and Powell recognize the power of the family when they characterize families as nurturing systems. This book deals with family support across the life span and within different settings. It prescribes new and more collaborative-oriented ways for practitioners to work with families. The purpose of the book is to refine and extend existing knowledge about approaches to supporting the caregiving roles of families across the life span.

Wasik, Barbara Hanna. 1990. *Home visiting.* Newbury Park, Calif.: Sage (304 pp.).

> *Home Visiting* represents one of the first modern attempts to present comprehensive information about procedures and issues related to home visiting with families. The author includes chapters on home visiting programs, personnel issues in home visiting, helping skills and techniques, visiting families in stressful situations, professional issues for home visitors, and future directions in home visiting.

Zarit, Steven H.; Leonard I. Pearlin; and K. Warner Schaie, eds. 1993. *Caregiving systems: Formal and informal helpers.* Hillsdale, N.J.: Lawrence Erlbaum Associates (332 pp.).

The authors address the topic of informal systems of care from a cultural perspective, considering the complexity of cultural contexts and their effect on care. The section on formal systems of care focuses on social health maintenance organizations and related public policy, home care services, barriers to use of services, and other related issues.

LOSS AND GRIEF

Bozarth, Alla R. 1986. *Life is goodbye, life is hello: Grieving well through all kinds of loss.* Minneapolis, Minn.: Compcare (203 pp.).

This author has guided others through all kinds of loss and disappointment: separation and change, physical death, death of a relationship, and even the death of a dream. Bozarth shows how to make grieving an action and helps readers become agents in their own healing process rather than victims of their grief.

Bozarth, Alla R. 1990. *A journey through grief.* Center City, Minn.: Hazelden (51 pp.).

In the long and anguishing journey of grief after the loss of a loved one, Dr. Alla R. Bozarth sensitively brings a message of assurance, comfort, and hope. Dr. Bozarth will tell you what to expect, what to do, and what to think. She will help you understand the physical symptoms of grieving and express what the loss really means to you.

Doka, Kenneth J., ed. 1995. *Children mourning, mourning children.* Washington, D.C.: Hospice Foundation of America (179 pp.).

This compassionate guide addresses the sensitive topic of children and grief. Death, life-threatening illness, and mourning are discussed from a child's perspective. Strategies for answering children's questions and talking to children about illness are included. The final section explains research in the field of children and grief and provides information about literature for children on death, dying, and bereavement.

Doka, Kenneth J., ed. 1996. *Living with grief after sudden loss.* Washington, D.C.: Hospice Foundation of America (271 pp.).

This book is the outgrowth of the 1996 teleconference "Living with Grief after Sudden Loss," sponsored by the Hospice Foundation of America. The articles contained in this text will help professional caregivers give aid to families dealing with loss, grief, and death. (It will also be beneficial to family members who have experienced the death of a loved one.) This book is specifically aimed at sudden loss, but anyone experiencing bereavement from any type of loss would be helped by some of the articles.

Kennedy, Alexandra. 1991. *Losing a parent: Passage to a new way of living.* San Francisco: Harper (139 pp.).

Losing a Parent offers readers an array of suggestions and techniques that will enable them to deal more effectively with the grief that a loved one's death causes. The author guides readers through this intense life change, providing help for gaining insight and maintaining inner peace.

Lewis, C. S. 1961. *A grief observed.* New York: HarperCollins (80 pp.).

A Grief Observed is a compilation of short journal-like entries that were written by a man mourning the loss of his wife. Writing this small book became "a defense against total collapse, a safety valve," and the author came to realize that "bereavement is a universal and integral part of our experience of love." This volume will help anyone who is dealing with grief and loss.

Livingston, Gordon. 1995. *Only spring: On mourning the death of my son.* New York: HarperCollins (230 pp.).

This journal was written by a father during the time his son was ill and dying and also after his death. It reveals the grief, helplessness, torment, hope, love, anguish, and strain the family experienced while coping with his illness and death. This is a book of survival of those who live on. It offers suggestions about how to grieve, gain strength, and confront great and difficult challenges in life.

Rando, Therese A. 1984. *Grief, dying, and death.* Champaign, Ill.: Research Press Company (476 pp.).

Early chapters of this book address the issues of bereavement, attitudes toward loss, reactions to loss, and unresolved grief, why these things occur, and how to work with individuals and families who are hurting from a loss. The latter half of the book looks at the issues of terminal illness care. Dr. Rando presents a sensitive but realistic approach to the difficult issues to be faced in the dying process. She offers many practical suggestions for the caregiver who is working with both individuals and families.

Rando, Therese A. 1986. *Parental loss of a child.* Champaign, Ill.: Research Press Company (555 pp.).

Parental loss of a child is unlike any other loss. The grief of parents is particularly severe, complicated, and long lasting, with major and unparalleled symptom fluctuations over time. Readable and insightful chapters discuss perspectives on the parental loss of a child, issues in specific types of death, socially unacknowledged parental bereavements, subjective experiences of death, professional help for bereaved parents, and organizations that can help.

Todd, Andrew, ed. 1995. *Journey of the heart: Stories of grief as told by nurses in the NICU.* 2d ed. Nashville: Vanderbilt University Medical Center (271 pp.).

This book has two distinct parts. Part 1, which is emotional and moving, relates the stories nurses tell about their work, experiences, knowledge, emotions, and insights as nurses in the newborn intensive care unit. Part 2 (appendixes) includes several helpful tools: a glossary, grief support and what is done for families, bereavement checklist and follow-up, what to say and not to say to families in their time of grief, and resources and organizations.

MENTAL ILLNESS

Depression

Berger, Diane, and Lisa Berger. 1991. *We heard the angels of madness: A family guide to coping with manic depression.* New York: Quill, William, Morrow (308 pp.).

Diane and Lisa Berger share both the intimate and inspiring story of how their family coped with Mark's manic-depressive illness and the valuable information they gathered about manic depression over the course of his treatment. Up-to-date facts on drugs, doctors, therapy, insurance, and other resources are included. The authors discuss how to identify the symptoms of manic depression and avoid a false diagnosis, which treatments work and which don't, and the emotional experience of a mother battling for the sanity and well-being of her child.

Kerns, Lawrence L. 1993. *Helping your depressed child: A reassuring guide to the causes and treatments of childhood and adolescent depression.* Rocklin, Calif.: Prima Publishing (284 pp.).

Dr. Kerns explains why children get depressed and outlines the role that a parent or teacher can play in helping a child deal constructively with these feelings. Also discussed are possible treatments for childhood depression—therapy, drug therapy, and hospitalization.

Klein, Donald F., and Paul H. Wender. 1993. *Understanding depression: A complete guide to its diagnosis and treatment.* New York: Oxford University Press (181 pp.).

The authors offer a definitive guide to depressive illness—its causes, course, and symptoms. They clarify the difference between depression (which is a normal emotion) and biological depression (which is an illness) and include several self-rating tests that readers can use to help determine whether they should seek psychiatric evaluation to establish if they have a biological depressive illness. Klein and Wender describe the symptoms of biological depression, how depressive illness can affect people's lives, and different types of treatment available.

General Topics

Esser, Aristide H., and Sylvia D. Lacey. 1989. *Mental illness: A homecare guide.* New York: John Wiley & Sons (263 pp.).

This book was written to increase awareness of home-care alternatives in psychiatric treatment of chronic emotional and mental problems. It serves as a guide to help families reach home-care treatment decisions more decisively and comprehensively while remaining flexible in exploring various kinds of therapies and community support services. The authors show families what criteria to use in selecting professional services and how to help design a treatment program, cope with unforeseen circumstances, ensure self-preservation, and assist their disturbed relatives or friends in living a productive and rewarding life. Practical and understandable step-by-step instructions are given for dealing with the day-to-day problems in the medical treatment and psychosocial education of the ill family member.

Hatfield, Agnes B. 1987. *Families of the mentally ill: Coping and adaptation.* New York: Guilford Press (336 pp.).

A number of aspects of coping and adaptation for families of the mentally ill are covered in this guide. It begins with a historical perspective of family caregivers, culture and mental illness, and a model of effective coping and moves on to a discussion of how families cope with mental illness. Behavioral manifestations, family responses, social support, and coping strategies are explored. New perspectives on service provision and research are also mentioned.

Hatfield, Agnes B. 1990. *Family education in mental illness.* New York: Guilford Press (211 pp.).

This book provides the curriculum and the methodology for an educational approach to helping families with a mentally ill relative. The author explores an understanding of the current cultural context for providing services to the mentally ill and an understanding of the people being helped. These concepts are developed along with the related concepts of family consultation and psychoeducation. Provided is a knowledge base from which family educators can select curriculum content based on what families express as their needs. Also established are basic principles of adult learning and guidelines for effective and efficient learning.

Lafond, Virginia. 1994. *Grieving mental illness: A guide for patients and their caregivers.* Toronto, Canada: University of Toronto Press (95 pp.).

This is a self-help book for anyone who has experienced the effects of mental illness as a sufferer, family member, friend, or caregiver. The author offers advice on how to move forward from a mental illness. She states, "By consciously grieving we can help bring healing and wholeness to our lives, resulting in new ways of coping, reduced stress, and greater self-esteem." Self-help exercises are included.

Rogg, Carla, and Oskar Rogg. 1994. *Georgia mental health sourcebook.* Atlanta: Care Solutions (177 pp.).

Georgia has taken the lead to improve service delivery for people with mental illness by restructuring its public mental health, mental retardation, and substance abuse system. This guide aids in the understanding of mental illnesses and includes information about services available in Georgia. Topics included are where to get help, types of mental illnesses, children and mental health issues, specific mental health concerns, legal and ethical issues, and available resources.

Ross, Jerilyn. 1994. *Triumph over fear: A book of help and hope for people with anxiety, panic attacks, and phobias.* New York: Bantam Books (296 pp.).

Jerilyn Ross overcame her own phobia to become one of the nation's leading authorities on anxiety disorders, panic attacks, and phobias. In this comforting and inspiring book, she offers facts and techniques that can bring relief in a matter of weeks, no matter how long one has been suffering. Through fascinating case histories, she explores the many faces of anxiety and introduces the step-by-step treatment plans that have worked for her patients.

Todd, Tracy. 1994. *Surviving and prospering in the managed mental health care marketplace.* Sarasota, Fla.: Professional Resource Press (85 pp.).

This book was written to help mental health care providers understand the current situation regarding their profession and to develop strategies for coping with legislative changes. Topics include understanding managed care systems, identifying and applying to provider networks, getting referrals, making adjustments as a therapist, impacted disciplines, the role of employee assistance programs, and questions and answers. Appendixes include a sample marketing letter, questions to ask the managed care system, a checklist for billing considerations, and sample managed care practice assessments.

Woolis, Rebecca. 1992. *When someone you love has a mental illness: A handbook for family, friends, and caregivers.* New York: Putnam Books (232 pp.).

This guide addresses daily problems of living with a person with mental illness, as well as long-term planning and care. Of special note are the forty-three "Quick Reference Guides" dealing with such topics as responding to hallucinations, delusions, violence, and anger; helping a loved one comply with treatment and medication plans; deciding where the person should live; and choosing a doctor. The book is intended to be used as a handbook by families and friends of people with mental illness to help them understand that person and how to deal with him or her day to day.

Schizophrenia

Anderson, Carol M.; Douglas J. Reiss; and Gerard E. Hogarty. 1986. *Schizophrenia and the family: A practitioner's guide to psychoeducation and management.* New York: Guilford Press (365 pp.).

The authors approach schizophrenia from a psychoeducational approach, taking into account the family's role as primary caretaker. The process of developing a productive treatment relationship with the patient and family is explored, and training issues and other applications of the psychoeducational model are addressed.

Backlar, Patricia. 1994. *The family face of schizophrenia*. New York: Jeremy P. Tarcher/Putnam (283 pp.).

Patricia Backlar, a mental health ethicist and mother of a son who suffers from schizophrenia, eloquently recounts true stories about families whose adult children suffer from this cruel disease. Following each narrative, experts from various mental health professions offer advice on the issues raised by each story. This book teaches readers how to navigate the complicated labyrinth of medical and social services and to become more effective in managing schizophrenia.

Torrey, E. Fuller. 1995. *Surviving schizophrenia: A manual for families, consumers, and providers*. 3d ed. New York: HarperCollins (409 pp.).

In clear language, this author describes the nature, causes, symptoms, treatment, and course of schizophrenia and also explores living with it from both the patient's and the family's point of view. This edition includes the latest research findings on what causes the disease as well as information about new drugs and offers answers to frequently asked questions.

MULTIPLE SCLEROSIS

Carroll, David L. 1993. *Living well with MS*. New York: HarperCollins (259 pp.).

Living Well with MS fills a strong need for a comprehensive book that will both comfort and inform the patient, family, and caregiver. The author carefully addresses topics such as diagnosis and prognosis, treatments for MS, exercises, diet, sexual dysfunction, emotional coping, and hope for a cure.

Kalb, Rosalind C., and Labe C. Scheinberg. 1992. *Multiple sclerosis and the family*. New York: Demos Publications (118 pp.).

This book includes discussions from experts in a variety of fields that explore the ways in which MS impacts the family group and describe strategies and resources that are available to help families manage their lives more effectively in the presence of MS. This volume will prove valuable to health care teams, professionals, and individuals with MS and their families.

PARKINSON'S DISEASE

Atwood, Glenna W. 1991. *Living well with Parkinson's: An inspirational and informative guide for Parkinsonians and their loved ones*. New York: John Wiley & Sons (198 pp.).

The author of this guide has Parkinson's disease and has risen to national prominence as a leading spokesperson for Parkinson's. She tells of her personal struggles with this tragic disease and offers new hope to others who must face it. Atwood describes her intimate, proven prescriptions for living well with Parkinson's, including up-to-date information and guidance. For example, an appendix/directory lists the kinds of special clothing and equipment available and where to get them.

Hutton, Thomas J., and Raye L. Pippel. 1989. *Caring for the Parkinson patient.* Buffalo, N.Y.: Prometheus Books (196 pp.).

This thoughtful collection of fourteen essays offers helpful information and useful suggestions relevant to virtually every concern voiced by parents, families, and caregivers. Experts in many fields contribute to provide information on topics such as new drug therapies, neural transplants, nursing techniques, exercises for movement and speech skills, how the disease impacts the family, and where to seek help when support is needed.

Katz, Richard. 1988. *Improving communication in Parkinson's disease.* Austin, Tex.: Pro-Ed (25 pp.).

The purpose of this booklet is to inform people about Parkinson's disease and to focus on one of its most common and painful problems, the breakdown in communication. It introduces and describes classic symptoms, speech characteristics, speech treatment, various types of difficulties and therapies, psychological considerations, and support groups and organizations.

PLANNING FOR THE FUTURE (FINANCIAL, LEGAL, EDUCATIONAL)

Berkobien, Richard. 1991. *A family handbook on future planning.* Arlington, Tex.: Association for Retarded Citizens of the United States (133 pp.).

This manual is a comprehensive source of information on planning the future for a loved one, especially one with a physical or mental disability. It includes making financial arrangements and writing a will and/or letter of intent; answers questions about education, employment, financial support, and residential programs for people with disabilities; and presents materials for planning for the future. Income, asset, trust, and will forms; addresses of places to send for materials; and checklists are included.

Cane, Michael Allan. 1995. *The five-minute lawyer's guide to estate planning.* New York: Dell (223 pp.).

This practical handbook answers questions every person has about personal estate issues. Caregivers often experience an added pressure to plan ahead carefully for the care and well-being of their care receivers. Some of the topics covered in this book include estate planning goals; wills, trusts, and life insurance; durable powers of attorney; joint tenancy with right of survivorship; gifts to and care of minor children; gift, estate, and inheritance taxes; and probate procedures.

Goldfluss, Howard E. 1994. *Living wills and wills.* New York: Wings Books (244 pp.).

Living Wills and Wills was written by Judge Goldfluss to help people make sure their wishes are followed when they can no longer state their own desires or after their death. Readers will find information on living wills, rights of a patient under the Patient Self-determination Act, wills and trusts, beneficiaries, probate, and living trusts and addresses and phone numbers of bar associations in each state. A sample will and forms for living wills, health care proxy, and durable powers of attorney are also included.

Russell, L. Mark; Arnold E. Grant; Suzanne M. Joseph; and Richard W. Fee. 1994. *Planning for the future: Providing a meaningful life for a child with a disability after your death.* Evanston, Ill.: American Publishing Co. (416 pp.).

Planning for the Future is full of practical ideas and important information. It is an essential guide to parents of children who have disabilities. The authors explain how to prepare a life plan, a letter of intent, and a special-needs trust, as well as how to maximize the child's government benefits, avoid probate, reduce estate taxes, and protect against the devastating costs of old age.

STROKE

Collins, Ellwyn K. 1992. *Unprepared!: A husband's story of coping with his wife's stroke.* Minneapolis, Minn.: Deaconess Press (195 pp.).

Unprepared! is especially helpful and meaningful for men who find themselves in caregiving roles. Collins relates his experiences of suddenly assuming housekeeping duties and caregiving responsibilities after his wife's stroke. Readers learn how he dealt with his emotions, with practical matters (he even includes recipes with added bits of humor), and with the health care system and providers.

Paullin, Ellen. 1988. *Ted's stroke: The caregiver's story.* Cabin John, Md.: Seven Locks Press (175 pp.).

A personal account written by the wife of a man who suffered a stroke. The book vividly recounts time spent in intensive care, therapy, convalescence, and day-to-day coping. One chapter is written by a physician who discusses what causes strokes, what happens physiologically when they occur, and prevention and reduction of one's risks of having a stroke.

SUPPORT/SELF-HELP GROUPS

Fradkin, Louise; Mirca Liberti; and Edward Madara. 1993. *Guide to starting a self-help support group for caregivers of the aged.* Levittown, Pa.: Children of Aging Parents (CAPS) (62 pp.).

This book was written to serve as a guide for persons interested in starting caregiver self-help support groups in their communities. It includes information on factors to consider before beginning, how to start and keep a group going, and what to do at meetings. Appendixes include information ranging from sample forms and discussion questions to information on resources. Also included are pages on a variety of elder-care topics that can be copied and used as handouts for group members.

Hill, Karen. 1987. *Helping you helps me: A guide book for self-help groups.* 2d ed. Ottawa, Ontario: Canadian Council on Social Development (no page numbers).

This is a practical guide to starting and maintaining a self-help group. Leadership, membership, recruitment, fund-raising, problem solving, and decision making are among the more than twenty topics covered.

Katz, Alfred H.; Hannah L. Hedrick; Daryl Holtz Isenberg; Leslie M. Thompson; Therese Goodrich; and Austin H. Kutscher, eds. 1992. *Self-help: Concepts and applications.* Philadelphia: Charles Press (308 pp.).

The authors take a look at the severity of the need for self-help groups in America today. Self-help is discussed as it applies to specific diseases and medical conditions such as AIDS, Alzheimer's disease, multiple sclerosis, hearing loss, cancer, and sudden infant death syndrome. The authors explore the need for cooperation between organized medicine and self-help groups in the future of health care. Included is an analysis of how empowerment of individuals, families, and groups is fostered by self-help participation. This book will be an important resource for both self-help group activists and professional providers.

Powell, Thomas J., ed. *Working with self-help.* Silver Spring, Md.: National Association of Social Workers (355 pp.).

This book is for persons interested in the self-help movement, either professionally or personally. Topics discussed include basic helping mechanisms common to different kinds of self-help programs, different types of self-help organizations, ways human service professionals can work with selected parts of the movement, clearinghouses, misuses of self-help, and use of self-help as an instrument for negotiating with professionals. Information is also provided on specific self-help groups and ways to enhance self-help activities in minority communities.

White, Barbara J., and Edward J. Madara, eds. 1992. *The self-help sourcebook: Finding and forming mutual aid self-help groups.* 4th ed. Denville, N.J.: Saint Clares–Riverside Medical Center (208 pp.).

This book is for individuals who are looking for a group to meet their special needs, professionals seeking an appropriate referral point for a client or information about a problem, academicians and researchers who want local or national self-help group contacts and information, policy makers at all levels of government, and media people seeking personal reactions to recent crises. It includes information about self-help clearinghouses, toll-free help lines, national self-help groups/organizations, resources for rare and genetic disorders, and information on the "how-tos" of starting and running local self-help groups.

Wuthnow, Robert. 1994. *Sharing the journey: Support groups and America's new quest for community.* Riverside, N.J.: Free Press (463 pp.).

The author reports on a definitive and illuminating study of the phenomenon of support groups in America. Wuthnow examines the growth of the support group movement and its meaning in our national life. *Sharing the Journey* illustrates how support groups develop, function, and serve the community. The possibilities and dangers of building community through support groups are explored. This book will provide new insights for anyone who wants to understand why small groups are a powerful source of identity in America today.

Contributors

PAM DAVIS received a B.A. in psychology and M.Ed. in behavioral science from Georgia Southwestern State University. She has completed additional graduate study in social work. Ms. Davis currently serves as assistant director of Middle Flint Behavioral HealthCare, a public mental health, mental retardation, and substance abuse program serving eight rural counties in southwest Georgia. She is a member of the Executive Committee of the West Central Georgia Caregivers Network (CARE-NET).

PAUL R. DOKECKI is professor of psychology and special education, a John F. Kennedy Center scholar, and a scholar at the Center for Clinical and Research Ethics at Vanderbilt University. He earned the Ph.D. in clinical psychology from George Peabody College in 1968. He is former editor of the *Peabody Journal of Education*. His scholarly interests include the philosophy of science, human science methodology, values and ethics, public policy, early childhood intervention for children with handicaps and their families, and community psychology intervention. His publications have appeared in a wide variety of journals, including the *Journal of Community Psychology, Infants and Young Children, Developmental Psychology,* and *Child Development.* His latest book, *The Tragi-Comic Professional,* was published in 1996 by Duquesne University Press.

JOHN J. GATES, Ph.D., is currently director of the mental health program at the Carter Center in Atlanta, where he supports the work of Rosalynn Carter and the Carter Center Mental Health Task Force. Dr. Gates serves on the boards of the Rosalynn Carter Institute for Human Development, the National Mental Health Association, and the World Federation for Mental Health. Previously, he was the Georgia state director of mental health, mental retardation, and substance abuse services.

DAVID HAIGLER, Ed.D., is deputy director of the Rosalynn Carter Institute of Georgia Southwestern State University. He is a licensed masters social worker (LMSW) in Georgia with more than twenty years of experience in mental health and human services. Dr. Haigler is coauthor of *Characteristics, Concerns, and Con-*

crete Needs of Formal and Informal Caregivers: Understanding and Appreciating Their Marathon Existence, issued in 1993 by Georgia Southwestern State University; and he is codeveloper of *Caring for You, Caring for Me: Education and Support for Caregivers.* He has conducted numerous caregiver education programs and professional presentations on caregiving.

KELLY NOSER HAYNES is a doctoral candidate at Vanderbilt University. She is working as an NIMH trainee at the Vanderbilt Institute for Public Policy in the Center for Mental Health Policy. Her current research efforts focus on assessing and improving the quality of mental health services.

ANNE G. MCWILLIAMS is a Ph.D. candidate in religion and personality at Vanderbilt University. She is currently a research assistant in the department of neurology at the University of Mississippi Medical Center. She has also been an adjunct instructor in the senior seminar of the University of Mississippi School of Medicine in the subject of ethics at the end of life. Her dissertation research is concerned with ethics in communication in pastoral care and counseling.

ROBERT M. MORONEY is professor of social policy and planning at the School of Social Work, Arizona State University. He is the author of eight books and more than fifty articles and book chapters on various aspects of policy, planning, and program evaluation. He has been associated with a number of policy institutes, including the Bush Institute at the University of North Carolina and the Vanderbilt Institute for Public Policy Studies. He currently serves as a board member of the Rosalynn Carter Institute for Human Development. Professor Moroney does extensive consultation with numerous national, state, and local human service agencies. He also recently was awarded a senior Fulbright award and was affiliated with University College, Dublin.

JOHN ROBERT NEWBROUGH is professor of psychology, human development, and special education and a John F. Kennedy Center scholar at Peabody College of Vanderbilt University. He received his doctoral degree from the University of Utah in 1959. In 1966, he joined the faculty of the Department of Psychology, George Peabody College for Teachers, Nashville, Tennessee, where he directs the Community Psychology program, and directed the Center for Community Studies, John F. Kennedy Center for Research on Education and Human Development, until 1980. He was editor of the *Journal of Community Psychology* from 1975 to 1990 and continues as editor emeritus responsible for special issues. His books include *Community Mental Health: A Reference Guide* and *Living Environments for Developmentally Retarded Persons.* He serves as a board member of the Rosalynn Carter Institute for Human Development. He is currently working on a theory of community called "The Third Position" to denote a move beyond the theory of the village and the theory of the city in an attempt to provide for understanding diversity in the postmodern world.

JACK A. NOTTINGHAM is the executive director of the Rosalynn Carter Institute, Georgia Southwestern State University. Dr. Nottingham has held professorships in psychology at the University of Maryland International Division, Western Michigan University, and the University of Hawaii. He is coeditor of the book *The Professional and Family Caregiver: Dilemmas, Rewards, and New Directions,* issued by Georgia Southwestern State University, and codeveloper of *Caring for You, Caring for Me: Education and Support for Caregivers.* Dr. Nottingham received his Ph.D. in psychology from George Peabody College of Vanderbilt University.

DAVID LEWIS SMITH is professor of sociology at Georgia Southwestern State University. He received his Ph.D. from the University of Tennessee in 1972. He has published numerous articles and book chapters in the areas of deviance and victimology. His current interest in caregiving focuses on measuring burnout in both informal and formal caregivers.

Index

Caregivers (*continued*)
caregiving experiences, 108–9; comparative ranking of needs with informal caregivers, 123; demographics, 108; importance of religion to, 122; inadequate educational opportunities for, 118; loss of idealism, 117; professional growth, 117; reasons for career choice, 109–10; reluctance to seek counseling, 121; rewards of caregiving, 116

Caregivers, informal (lay or family): adaptation process, 65; barriers to service use by, 68–69; centrality of, to caregiving process, 55, 66; defined, 103; empowerment, 96–101; information needs, 57–58; lost income, 61; need for organization, 89, 99–100; need for respite, 61; provision of assistance with activities of daily living, 58–59; provision of financial support, 61

Caregivers, informal (lay or family), in CARE-NET study: advice for formal caregivers, 120; amount of time spent in caregiving, 110, 112; anxiety about changes in caregiving situation, 114; attitudes toward formal caregivers, 119, 120; burnout, 121–22; caregiving alternatives available to, 114; comparative ranking of needs with formal caregivers, 123; degree of choice in caregiving role, 115–16; demographics, 110; differences caregiving made in lives, 117–18; duration of caregiving experience, 111; importance of religion to, 122; inadequate communication with formal caregivers, 119; inadequate educational opportunities for, 118; kinds of caregiving assistance provided, 111–12; lack of adequate alternatives for caregiving, 114–15; nature of problem requiring care, 110; negative impact of caregiving on financial and employment situations, 115; range of resources used, 113; reluctance to seek counseling, 121; rewards and burdens of caregiving, 115–

16; sources of moral support, 113–14; support available, 112–13

Caregivers, volunteer, 103–4

Caregiving, 1, 100; approach to, from 1970s on, 20–21; approach to, from 1930s to 1970s, 19–20; barriers to, 64, 72–78; as caring, 7; and communicative claims, 48–49; and competing role demands, 52; defined, 2; either-or thinking regarding best system of, 37; exploitation in, 9–10; interdependency of formal and informal systems of, 37–38; and partnership and shared responsibility, 44–45; proposed solutions to barriers, 79–82; roles, 53; services in, 54; and stress, 50–53

Caregiving, formal system, 2; barriers within, 41–44; guidelines for service provision, 73; need for choice in, 74–75; role and functions of, 55; shift from pathology-based to wellness models, 82; view of, as sum total of service components, 74

Caregiving, informal system, 2; centrality of, to caregiving process, 55, 66; decreased resources for, in times of retrenchment, 4; provision of, by women, 33–34; shift in ratio of caregiving women to elderly, 34; trend away from, 3

Caregiving professions: reasons for entering, 9, 109–10

Caregiving service delivery: changes in, to increase consumer satisfaction, 97–98; choice as basis of, 73; discontinuity of, 77–78; fragmentation of, 75–76; inaccessibility of, 76–77; lack of accountability of, 78; reform proposals, 79–82, 83–86

Caregiving services: emotional/cognitive, 56, 57, 62–65; instrumental, 56, 57–62

Caregiving services integration, 79–82; challenges to implementation of, 87

CARE-NET needs assessment study: characteristics of formal caregivers, 108–10, 116–23; characteristics of informal care-

Medicaid, 28, 62

Medicare, 62

Mentally disabled persons: estimated number of, 28; legal issues as barrier to caregiving, 77

Mental retardation, profound, 9, 10

Model Cities, 79, 96

Moroney, R. M., 45

Mothers, shift from caretaking of children to elderly, 33

Mullan, J. T., 51, 61, 68

Nagi, S., 27

National Alliance for the Mentally Ill, 98

National Family Caregivers Association (NFCA), 99

National Mental Health Consumer Association, 98

National Quality Caregiving Coalition (NQCC), 99

Needs assessment, 17, 79, 105

Nottingham, J., 60, 63

Oken, D., 61, 63

Old Age Survivors Disability Insurance (OASDI), 62

Osborne, D., 83–84

Parker, G., 7

Participatory decision making, and caring, 16–17

Partnership, 44–45

Pathology-based models, 82

Patience, as ingredient of caring, 12

Penrod, J. D., 58

Performance measurement, 86, 89

Performance Partnership Grants (PPGs), 86

Personal projects, 47

Poor Law, 20, 25

Power: directive, 46; professional, 45–47; synergic, 46–47

Problem-focused services, 56

Problem setting, 41

Problem solving, 41

"Profamily" movement, 23

Professional caregivers. *See* Caregivers, formal (professional)

Professional education, 94–96

Professional myopia, 76

Professional power, 45–47

Professional roles, models of: reflective practice (Model II), 42, 43, 44, 94, 95, 100; technical rationality (Model I), 41–42, 43, 44

Professions, crisis of, 41

Projection, 65

Psychotherapy, 64–65

Public health nurses, 91–92

Purchase of service contracting (POSC), 84–85; likely effect on informal caregivers, 88

Rain Man (film), 40

Reflective practice (Model II), 42, 43, 44, 94, 95, 100

Reflective Practitioner, The (Schön), 41–42, 43, 67, 80, 127 (chap. 3, n. 2)

Regarding Henry (film), 40

Reinventing Government (Osborne and Gaebler), 83–84

Residual approach, to social policy, 21

Residual means tested program, 62

Resource allocation, 79

Resource constraints, 72–75

Respite, 60–61

Richardson, Eliot, 79

Richmond, J. B., 64–65

Riley, L., 27

Rosalynn Carter Institute: and CARE-NET Study, 105, 106; National Quality Caregiving Coalition (NQCC), 99; study of caregiving, 78, 127 (n. 2)

Rosenbaum, Ed, 39

Sarason, Seymour B., 1

Schön, Donald, 41–42, 43, 67, 80, 127 (chap. 3, n. 2)

Schorr, A., 36

Schreiber, L., 39–40